It's Not About the Broccoli

· · ·

Three Habits to Teach Your Kids for a Lifetime of Healthy Eating

· · ·

Dina Rose, PhD

A PERIGEE BOOK

A PERIGEE BOOK
Published by the Penguin Group
Penguin Group (USA) LLC
375 Hudson Street, New York, New York 10014

USA • Canada • UK • Ireland • Australia • New Zealand • India • South Africa • China

penguin.com

A Penguin Random House Company

Library of Congress Cataloging-in-Publication Data

Rose, Dina.
It's not about the broccoli : three habits to teach your kids for a lifetime
of healthy eating / Dina Rose, PhD.— First edition.
pages   cm
Includes bibliographical references.
ISBN 978-0-399-16418-7 (pbk.)
1. Children—Nutrition.   2. Natural foods.   3. Health promotion.   I. Title.
RJ206.R668   2014
613.2083—dc23   2013033502

First edition: January 2014

PRINTED IN THE UNITED STATES OF AMERICA

10 9 8 7 6 5 4 3 2

In loving memory of my mother,
who tried her hardest to give me the tools for
a better "food life," and for my daughter,
my inspiration and delight.

CONTENTS

It's Not About the Broccoli

Part One

• • •

Bagels, Pizza, Pasta, Nuggets

How Did We Get Here?

Why It's Not About the Broccoli

When I was five months pregnant, my mother died. She was sixty-five years old and weighed just over three hundred pounds. Although she had not been obese for her entire life, she had struggled with her weight ever since I could remember. Food was her obsession, her frenemy, and her distraction from pain. It was her lifeline as well as the noose around her neck. While I may never know the extent to which my mother's overeating caused her death, I do know it caused her years of distress.

Although my mother tried to protect me from her demons, quite a few of them transferred down to me: a poor body image, out-of-control snacking, and, more often than I care to admit, a ravenous desire for sweets. When my daughter was born, I was painfully aware that I wanted my child to have a better "food life." I wanted her to be able to nourish herself *and* have a happy relationship with food.

Many of my friends had the same goals. Like me, they didn't always have the easiest time eating right. Some had grown up with too much junk. Others were forced to clean their plates. And many of us learned to comfort ourselves with cookies. As adults, we all worked hard to approach food differently. We read books about nutrition and health; we sought out healthy recipes; we even ate our vegetables! What's more, we tried not to go diving for the ice cream at the first sign of stress.

When we had families of our own, we told ourselves we wanted our children to eat well from the beginning. Of course we wanted good nutrition for them. Although experts don't always agree on the best way to feed kids, we could easily discern the basics: Kids need fresh, wholesome foods, including fruits and vegetables, quality protein, and whole grains, along with milk or some other source of calcium. But we wanted more for our children. We wanted them to know the difference between physical and emotional hunger, to be able to stop *before* they'd devoured the entire bag of chips. We also wanted them to try all kinds of foods—Mexican, Indian, Japanese, Thai!—so they could join us on *our* food adventures.

But I noticed that when my friends actually had kids of their own, something changed. The parents were shocked, then flattened, by how hard it was to feed their families well. Some of them even described their family's food struggles in the language of combat: "Dinnertime is a war zone." "We are waving the white flag on whole grains." "We are going to wrestle some calcium into Ethan if it kills us all."

Mealtimes were stressful events, with parents begging their children to eat and the children whining and rejecting their parents' entreaties. Over the years, it was easy to predict what most of these kids would end up eating at any given meal: pizza, noodles, chicken nuggets, or bagels, along with a fruit juice or sweetened drink. If food really was a battle, it was clear that the parents were losing.

Despite their lofty intentions, most of the parents I knew were raising their children to be picky, chicken-finger-lovin', emotional eaters who saw food as an arena for conflict and resistance. This was precisely the situation we'd all wanted to avoid. What had happened, and how could I prevent this misery around my own table?

How do you teach children to eat right? I was consumed with figuring this out. Because I'm a sociologist, I was naturally oriented to thinking more about how parents shape their children's behavior than about nutrition. But when I started studying this question, I discovered something I wasn't prepared for, something surprising. In fact, it was completely counterintuitive: The more that parents focus on nutrition, the worse their kids are likely to eat.

I discovered something else, too: There's an alternative to the nutrition mindset, one that—ironically—is more effective at teaching kids to become healthy eaters. It's an alternative that parents describe as both doable and revolutionary. But I'm getting ahead of myself. To explain, I need to tell you a little more about myself and about my unusual perspective on food and eating.

HABITS AND HEALTHY EATING

When my daughter started eating solids, I used the tools of my profession, sociology, to teach her how to eat right. Back then, I was working in criminology; my research focused on families living in high-crime neighborhoods. In particular, I looked at how families sometimes managed to raise their children to become law-abiding citizens even when everything in their immediate environment was working against them. Other sociologists I know examined things like how marriage choices affect children or how kids learn about gender roles. But one of the key concepts that ties all these topics together is socialization: how groups of people—families included—pass on their values and behaviors to the next generation and how children repeat those behaviors until they become habits. (In sociology speak, we think of habits as behaviors that become so routine we do them without thinking about it.)

When I eventually left my work as a criminologist so that I could turn my attention full time to the topic of how parents teach their kids to eat right, a lot of my friends joked that I was studying the same subject as in my old university days: how to get deviants to do the right thing! It was funny, but it also had the ring of truth. That's because so many of our actions are shaped by the lessons we learn, consciously and subconsciously, from our families. Those lessons translate into behaviors (both good and bad), and over time, those behaviors become habits. That's the process, and it doesn't matter whether we're talking about criminals or kids! We are free to make our own choices, of course, but as we all know, it's hard to break a habit once it's formed.

Because of my background, I didn't think about feeding my daughter in terms of food—as crazy as that sounds. I thought about it in terms of the lessons I would teach her and the habits she would subsequently learn. With my attention firmly fixed on habits, I looked around and started seeing lessons and habits everywhere. If I was at a friend's house and broccoli was served, for example, I paid attention to what the parents said to their kids about the broccoli. Did the parents feel they had to get their kids to eat the broccoli by any means necessary, and if they did, what happened? If the child used his spoon as a catapult to launch the broccoli across the kitchen, how did the parents respond? I looked at the kind of eating environment the parents created. Was it happy and relaxed, or was it tense? And above all, I wondered what the children were learning from these interactions. Were they learning to fight about food, or were they learning the kinds of habits that would help them grow into teenagers and adults who willingly ate vegetables? Were they learning how to excitedly explore new foods? How to easily get through buffets, holidays, and other eating extravaganzas without overdoing it?

Habits can sound a lot like etiquette: putting your napkin on your lap, chewing with your mouth closed, and knowing which fork to use. Some people use the term *habits* to mean other manners, such as eating at the table or in front of the television. But the habits I was thinking about are the ones that reflect what we are accustomed to eating and that affect what we'll choose to eat in the future.

Kids develop lots of eating habits, and they do it very early on. Some habits are obvious. If your child always drinks milk first thing in the morning or always insists on snacking from the same *Backyardigans* bowl, it is clearly a habit. Other habits are more subtle: When kids insist on eating a diet of peanut butter and jelly sandwiches, hot dogs, and chicken nuggets (but only that *one* particular brand that they like), that's a habit. When they skimp on meals and then demand snacks, that's a habit. When kids say, "I don't like it," before they've even taken a taste, that's a habit, too.

For better or worse, children carry their eating habits with them into later life. True, most children eventually move beyond PB&J and hot dogs, but the basic habit of eating a limited, repetitive diet, without a lot of fruits and vegetables, often stays the same. But even if kids do change their habits as they grow up, what then? Those changes will take a lot of hard work, both for you *and* for them. When it comes to your own diet, don't you just know that it would be easier to eat the way you want to now if you had formed different habits from the get-go? Habits such as snacking on fruit and not eating once you're full? Of not rewarding yourself with treats when you've had a hard day? I know I'd like to be able to have just one (OK, just *two*) cookies when I break out the box.

I realized that if I were going to end my family's cycle of mothers passing bad eating habits down to their children, I would have to be very conscious of the lessons I taught my daughter. Have you seen parents scrape the last bits of baby cereal out of a bowl and say to their child, "Come on, one more bite. You can do it!" Well, the first thing I decided was that my daughter would be in charge of her own tummy. I wasn't going to tell her when she was done eating—*she* would always tell *me*. I hoped this would help her avoid the habit of overeating, the habit that had caused my mother—her grandmother—so much pain.

A lot of people avoid giving their babies sugar for the first year. Their goal is to prevent their child from developing a sweet tooth. Because I knew firsthand that oversnacking leads to overeating, I took a similar line against prepackaged snack foods. Instead of regularly giving my daughter crackers and cookies at snack time, I typically gave her soft fruits and vegetables. I wanted to prevent my daughter from developing a preference for the very salty or sweet snacks that are the downfall of so many diets.

To many people, my habits approach seemed bizarre. "She's just a baby!" they said. Or, "Are a couple of cookies really going to hurt her?" But to me, the habits approach made perfect sense. I wasn't thinking about the food; I was thinking about the bigger lesson that those foods were teaching. If I didn't teach those lessons now, when else would my daughter learn them? If I wasn't (mostly) consistent, how would my lessons be clear?

One day, when my daughter was around eight months old, we were in the park. Another mother started handing out cookies to all the kids. When I explained that I didn't want my daughter to have a cookie, that I'd brought fruit for her instead, the woman responded, "But this is OK; it's Gerber." At that point, I realized there was a very big gap between how this woman saw the eating world and how I saw it. She saw a cookie that didn't have any bad stuff, like sugar, in it. I didn't really see the cookie. I saw the lesson that my daughter would learn: That crunchy cookies are more fun than fruit. A lot of parents seemed to think that it was crazy to try to teach children these lessons at a young age. But because childhood, even babyhood, is when it all starts, that's the time to get good habits in place. Of course, as my daughter grew up, I started giving her cookies and even cake, ice cream, and candy. But by then she understood that these were exceptions and not the everyday way of eating.

THE NUTRITION MINDSET: HOW GOOD PARENTS TEACH BAD EATING HABITS

My habits approach seemed to be working at home. I adjusted and broadened it as my daughter grew, but I always kept my gaze fixed firmly on the long-term prize. And now, twelve years later, she does not overeat. She snacks mostly on healthy food, and when she does have a treat like a brownie, she can take a few bites and, if she's full, *walk away*. She's an adventurous eater who loves to try new foods. She even decided to become a vegetarian, and not the kind who lives on foods like pasta and cheese. She actually eats vegetables!

But from a professional standpoint, I was hooked: Criminology faded from my radar. Instead, I was now driven to know more about how parents and their children interacted around food and how eating habits were created. It wasn't long before I was engaged in a full-blown investigation. In addition to observing parents, I delved into the scientific literature in nutrition, food psychology, sociology, and parenting; I thought more about the process of socialization; I formulated theories. Then I started interviewing parents, sometimes one on one and sometimes in small groups. I wanted to know how these parents thought about the job of feeding their kids. I asked people whether they were happy with their kids' diets, what aspects they wished were different, and why they thought they were having the problems they were having. Then I asked them *what* they fed their children and, most important, *why*. I wanted to know if they were thinking about habits. And that's how I discovered the mother of all ironies: The more that parents focus on nutrition, the worse their kids tend to eat.

I'm sure you will recognize the problems most of the parents I interviewed were having. Their kids didn't eat a lot of fast food or candy, but like the children I'd observed years before, they ate diets that were predictably limited to just a couple of fruits and vegetables, plenty of sweets, and lots of mediocre fare like mac 'n' cheese, hot dogs, bagels, and chicken nuggets. In some families, there was plenty of conflict over food (some of the parents clearly dreaded mealtimes with the kids). Other families characterized their children's diets as OK. They wished their children would eat better, but without knowing how to change things, they had reached an impasse that everyone in the family seemed to find acceptable.

I wasn't surprised that so many of the parents I interviewed were struggling to feed their kids well. Most American kids eat poorly:

- On any given day, 30 percent of all two- to three-year-olds don't eat a single vegetable. Yet almost every preschooler in the country consumes some type of sweetened beverage, dessert, or sweet or salty snack on a daily basis.

- When children do eat vegetables, french fries are the vegetable they're most likely to eat.

- Nearly 40 percent of the total calories consumed by two- to eighteen-year-olds are in the form of empty calories, far exceeding the recommended allowance for discretionary calories. On average, children reach for cookies, chips, and other snacks three times a day.

- Some researchers worry that children are moving to a near constant state of eating by consuming either snacks or meals as often as ten times a day.

- The Centers for Disease Control and Prevention (CDC) reports that approximately 17 percent (or 12.5 million) of children and adolescents aged two to nineteen years are obese. Since 1980, the prevalence of obesity among children and adolescents has almost tripled.

- About 25 percent of overweight children aged five to seventeen years have two or more risk factors for cardiovascular disease, including high cholesterol levels, high blood pressure, and abnormal glucose tolerance.

- Children today have a 30 percent chance of developing diabetes during their lifetime.

Scientists predict that today's children may be the first in U.S. history to have a shorter life expectancy than their parents. Why? Because bad eating habits don't disappear as children grow up; they get worse. Compared to preschoolers, elementary school children are almost *three times* more likely to underconsume fruit, and *one and half times* more likely to underconsume vegetables. High schoolers are *four times* more likely to underconsume fruit than preschoolers and nearly *two and half times* more likely to underconsume vegetables.

When most nutrition experts look at the data on how poorly kids eat, they blame food manufacturers, television advertising, school lunch programs, and fast-food restaurants—and it's clear to me that all these factors play a role in how kids eat. It's hard to teach children to eat right when there's so much questionable food out there and so many messages designed to convince parents to serve it and kids to eat it.

When these same experts look at families, however, they come to the conclusion that parents don't pay *enough* attention to nutrition. Yet most of the struggling parents I interviewed were fluent in the language of nutrition and nutrients. They talked a lot about calcium, fat, and sugar. They knew about antioxidants and omega-3 fatty acids. In short, they knew what their kids *ought* to eat. On the other hand, although the parents thought a lot about nutrition, when I asked them about the long-term lessons (or habits) they wanted to teach their children, they stumbled a bit to find an answer. "Eat fruits and vegetables?" they'd say tentatively. It was clear that most parents hadn't really thought about this. So many parents fit this pattern that I gave it a name: *the nutrition mindset.*

Don't get me wrong, kids need healthy foods; it's just that when it comes to teaching kids how to eat well, the nutrition mindset—in which the parents focus tightly on the nutrients that their children are eating—isn't very effective. That's because most parents who have the nutrition mindset live in a state of quasi-panic about the nutrients their kids do or do not eat. The consequences of failing to get the right nutrition seem enormous to them. On its own, this belief makes feeding kids stressful. But the nutrition mindset comes with a couple of other beliefs that make the situation worse and, ultimately, lead kids to develop habits that are the opposite of the ones their parents would like them to have.

For example, parents with the nutrition mindset typically subscribe to a popular belief that kids are either good eaters or not, and there's nothing you can do about it. Closely related to this belief is the idea that it's unreasonable to expect children to like healthy foods. Never mind that it's pretty easy to debunk the kids-need-to-eat-child-friendly-foods myth. After all, Indian kids eat Indian food, and Mexican kids eat Mexican food; they don't eat hot dogs and chicken nuggets. In this country, however, we believe that kids like bland and beige food. And they definitely don't like vegetables.

Now, the parents I know would agree with the general sentiment that most children will end up liking a wider array of foods . . . eventually. But that's long-term thinking. The nutrition mindset promotes short-term thinking; it focuses parents' attention on the immediate meal, sometimes even on the immediate mouthful. That puts parents in a bind: How do you get kids to consume nutrients *today* when you know they don't like nutritious foods?

For parents with the nutrition mindset, the solution is obvious. The next chapter describes this solution in greater detail, so I'll give it just a brief description here. You search around for foods that meet two criteria: They pass the nutrition sniff test (that is, they have at least one or two nutrients that you can feel good about), and your kids will eat them. These criteria lead well-intentioned parents to serve kid-friendly foods like mac 'n' cheese (it has calcium), hot dogs (they have protein), and bagels (they're fat free). Then they offer these same few foods day in and day out because doing so minimizes the struggle and gets the job done. Do you see some habits forming here?

The problem with this kind of diet, aside from the obvious drawback that it's not very good for you, is that it sets off a chain reaction; kids' taste buds become accustomed to these extremely fatty, salty, and sweet foods (those preferences are a habit), and *that* makes them more inclined to reject fresh foods that don't have the same flavor kick (another habit). To get their kids to drink plain milk or to eat broccoli, parents resort to pressure tactics: They cheer, they wheedle, they command, they threaten, and they bribe.

("There are brownies for dessert!") No parent I know wants to use these strategies, but when getting nutrients into your kids feels like a task you *have* to do, you do what has to be done.

Unfortunately, pressuring children to eat foods they don't want to eat makes them less likely to want to eat those foods. How many of the foods that you were forced to eat during your childhood do you really enjoy eating today? But the pressure dynamic does something more, something even worse: It turns you and your kids into adversaries. *That* sets the stage for a massive control struggle.

Parents with the nutrition mindset also tend to have some ways of parenting—you can think of these as parenting habits or even parenting hang-ups—that make it hard for them to set boundaries and to parent their children consistently around food and eating. Some habitually avoid conflict; others habitually give their kids food as a way to tamp down uncomfortable emotions. Again, when you mix these hang-ups with the need to get *enough* of the *right* nutrients into kids *today*, you have a recipe for problems. (For more about these hang-ups—and we've all got them—see Chapter 3.)

Because so many of us have the nutrition mindset, parents look around and see families with the same kinds of problems they have. Those problems eventually seem unavoidable, even normal. Yet no one I know gives up. Parents continue to search for ways to get their kids to eat better.

Some try taking a zero-tolerance stance, like one woman I know. When her children refused to eat the lasagna she had prepared, she served it at every meal for a week. "That'll teach them," she said. Controlling, high-pressure tactics like these may—sometimes—silence the whining and quiet the battles. But they result in kids who feel bitter about the eating experience and who don't know how to make good choices later in life.

Others try grocery shopping with their children, cooking with them, or planting a garden. All these activities are great and some-times work. But if they haven't worked for you, it's probably be-cause they can't counteract the undesirable effects of the nutrition mindset. Every drop of positive change produced by cooking to-gether on Sunday night, for instance, is easily overwhelmed by the bucket of negative consequences that come from serving kids a steady stream of child-friendly foods all the rest of the time. Some experts tell parents that they should model what to eat, to let kids "catch" them eating well. Of course, you can't expect your kids to eat fish if you're eating fries, but modeling is too passive to create the kind of major turnaround that parents are looking for. Imagine that you and your child are fighting constantly over what to wear to school, and someone tells you that the best way to teach your kids to get dressed in the mornings is to teach them to sew or to let them catch you wearing nice clothes. Modeling simply isn't powerful enough to make lasting change if the underlying feeding dynamic is constantly working against you.

But even if modeling does increase vegetable consumption, what then? Would you really call a gaggle of kids who eat their peas—happily, winningly, and with gusto—healthy eaters if they also ha-bitually eat way too many cookies and doughnuts? If they turn to snacks when they're bored? If they throw a tantrum when new foods hit their plates? Kids need more than a model; they need in-struction on these habits, too.

The nutrition mindset is a trap. It encourages parents to evaluate the merits of individual foods, on individual days and at individual meals, and to overlook the broader patterns and underlying lessons their kids are learning. Moreover, the nutrition mindset teaches children a distinctly American attitude about food: Healthy food tastes bad; it's eaten for health, not for pleasure; eating healthy food earns us the right to indulge in junk food; and the junkier some-

Never Before Has a Nation Known So Much About Nutrition, Yet Eaten So Poorly

It takes surprisingly little knowledge about nutrition to eat right. Recently, a collaborative team of French, Canadian, and American researchers asked people in their respective countries to estimate the percentage of total fat in a list of foods such as butter, milk, margarine, and olive oil. Among the people who thought they could estimate the percentage of fat in different foods, the American respondents were most likely to be correct, and the French were most likely to be wrong. In fact, the French are a whopping ten times more ignorant than Americans on the question of dietary fats.

You know the punch line: The French are a nation of slim, trim, vegetable eaters who are generally healthy, and we're . . . not. The obesity rate in the United States is almost *three* times higher than it is in France.

What can explain these findings? The researchers concluded that in America it's easy to lose sight of the big picture because people have become consumers of nutrients instead of food, and the nutrient approach often results in questionable food choices.

thing is, the better it tastes. Research shows that this attitude stays with children forever.

WHAT SUCCESSFUL PARENTS DO

Fortunately there is encouraging news, too. Not everyone is struggling. A small group of parents I interviewed took a different approach to eating. These parents were focused on the long-term goal of raising healthy eaters, and by and large, they succeeded. Their children ate a wider range of healthy foods, they didn't whine for treats, and they were willing to try new textures and flavors.

How did this group produce better habits? By doing the unexpected. They didn't concentrate so much on nutrition—at least nutrition wasn't their primary orientation. They definitely weren't as scared as the other parents about what might happen if their children didn't take in enough of the right nutrients on any particular day. This freed them to worry less about how to get their kids to eat one more green bean *right now* and to think more about their long-term goal of raising children who made healthy choices. They recognized that eating, much like sleeping or bathing or manners, was an area that required a heavy dose of parental teaching. They set clear boundaries but were flexible enough to respond to their child's temperament and individual needs. They talked to their children about their goals. They were patient; they knew they were planting seeds of learning that might take weeks, months, or even longer to bloom. I came to label this style *the teaching approach*.

When their kids rejected certain foods, parents who used the teaching approach weren't flustered. It didn't seem like such a big deal to them, because they didn't buy into the myth that kids can't like healthy foods, and they weren't scared by nutrition consequences. This kept them from caving in and serving a steady diet of kid-friendly foods. When I asked one woman who used the teaching approach what she did when her kids didn't like what she served, she shrugged. "I wait a little while and then I serve it again," she said. She knew, instinctively, that kids will say they hate a food one day and like it the next. She didn't take their food rejection too seriously, but she didn't pressure her kids, either. She let her children pick and choose from the foods she served, but she stuck to her

Before You Begin

Nearly all kids suffer from garden-variety picky eating at one time or another. Some children have mild cases, and others are severely restricted in what they will eat, but when parents change the family's food behaviors, their children's eating improves.

In a few cases, though, a child's picky eating has a physical cause. The mechanics of eating seem simple when in fact they are fairly complicated, and some kids struggle with one of the steps: chewing, swallowing, digesting, or managing the sensory input that occurs when eating. These problems can be caused by oral–motor, sensory, postural, or developmental issues.

How do you spot a problem? Frequent gagging or vomiting (for reasons unrelated to illness), copious drooling, difficulty chewing, frequent constipation or diarrhea, a rigid preference for a particular food texture, and strong, persistent emotional reactions to food are signs that picky eating may have an underlying cause. Kids who lag behind developmental milestones in general may also have trouble eating. If your child has these symptoms or if your parental instinct tells you that something isn't right, have an evaluation performed.

Start by checking in with your child's pediatrician, but know that some parents have found it useful to consult an occupational or speech therapist. The American Speech-Language-Hearing Association (ASHA) lists therapists by city and state. Visit ASHA's website at asha.org. The book *Just Take a Bite: Easy, Effective Answers to Food Aversions and Eating Challenges!* by Lori Ernsperger and Tania Stegen-Hanson, is also a good reference for information about feeding problems and how to manage them.

plans to serve *real* food. She stayed relaxed, and over time, her kids did develop a taste for the good stuff.

Although they wouldn't have used sociology terms to describe what they were doing, the parents using the teaching approach wanted to create good habits: the habits of eating well and the habits of good parent–child interaction at snacks and mealtimes. They recognized that good eating habits don't just come from knowing what to eat. They come from knowing when, why, and how much to eat, too. So they devoted a lot of effort to setting structures for meals and snacks. They offered fresh, healthy meals and didn't prepare kid-friendly alternatives. They wanted their kids to develop the habit of being open to trying new foods; they weren't as inclined to push kids to eat one more bite. And when problems did arise, these parents reacted calmly. They didn't punish, and they didn't beg. They asked themselves, as good educators do, "What does my child need to learn to get past this rough spot?" Sometimes this meant teaching their children to accept new textures. Sometimes it meant defusing a control struggle.

Sound good? It did to me, too. Suddenly, my investigation had more focus. By bringing together my training as a sociologist, my experiences as a mother (and as a daughter), and what I had learned in the interviews and through reading the scientific literature, what had started out as a set of vague theories was now developing into a rich and deep understanding of how children learn to eat. What's more, as I identified the basis for the problems parents were having, it became clear what the solutions were: to focus less on how much broccoli gets eaten and to focus more on a teaching approach—that is, on shaping the interactions that lead to good eating habits.

THE THREE HABITS: (ALMOST) ALL YOU NEED TO KNOW

One of the best aspects of the teaching approach is that *you already know how to do it*. You just have to start thinking about eating much in the same way most of us think about good manners, good hygiene, or getting dressed: a set of habits that have to be learned and practiced. Of course, it can be harder to teach healthy eating habits than it is to teach, say, taking baths. Eating feels more personal and more emotional; it's a touchier subject. It happens more frequently, too—for kids, usually five or six times day. And whereas you have to work at rejecting the cultural messages that say it's impossible to teach kids good eating habits, this is hardly ever an issue in the tub. Has another parent ever said to you, "Don't give him soap yet! He's not old enough to like being clean—just wait and he'll grow into it eventually, maybe"?

But for most of us, the hardest part about teaching eating habits is figuring out how to break down this complex subject into clear guidelines that our kids can understand. In truth, parents teach their children a lot about eating. It's just that they focus mostly on teaching the fundamentals of food—"This is an orange. It's a fruit. Fruit is healthy."—and how to master technical skills, such as using a fork and a spoon. We forget, however, to help our children learn how to make decisions about what, when, why, and how much to eat.

Again, this isn't so difficult when it comes to other good habits. We explain to our kids why, for example, they have to wear a raincoat in the rain or why they can't wear a bathing suit to a wedding. We do this not just to make sure that our kids know what to do but because we believe that when kids understand *why*, they'll more happily comply. That, and we hope in time our kids will begin to make more appropriate decisions on their own. We'd never plunk down a pair of rain boots and expect a young child to figure out when and how to use them. Why, then, do we think it's right to plunk down a plate of Brussels sprouts and simply hope for the best? I suspect it's because when we think of eating in terms of nutrition, the explanations seem far too complicated.

What parents need is a rain-boots style of explanation that they can apply to eating. Parents who adopt the teaching approach have a way to do this. They teach their children three basic eating habits:

• Proportion

• Variety

• Moderation

Proportion means consuming foods in proportion to their healthful benefits; it's the habit of eating fresh, wholesome foods more often than junky ones. *Variety* means eating different kinds of foods. And *moderation* is the habit of eating the right amount of foods—not too much and not too little. Together, the three habits translate good nutrition into behavior; it's almost impossible to follow them and not eat well. When you teach proportion, variety, and moderation, there's a lot less tension around the table. You don't have to worry so much about what your children eat on a particular day, and you don't obsess about a couple of particular nutrients, because the overall pattern produces healthy eating habits.

You may have never heard of these three habits, but successful parents teach these habits to their children even when they are unaware that this is what they are doing. Moreover, these are the behaviors that form the basis of the U.S. Department of Agriculture's (USDA's) former Food Pyramid and its replacement, the MyPlate eating plan. (Why couldn't the USDA have just told us about these three habits? It's advice along the lines of "a serving size for children between the ages of two and three consists of half an apple or thirty-two seedless grapes" that drives parents up a tree. Yet the USDA notes in its document "MyPyramid Food Guidance System Education Framework" that proportion, variety, and moderation "are not intended as direct consumer messages, but rather as a framework of ideas from which professionals can develop consumer messages and materials."

It's easy to think that children are too young to learn proportion, variety, and moderation, but that's the beauty of these habits: They are easy to streamline into simple statements that even young children can understand and follow.

- **Proportion.** We eat foods like fruits and vegetables more often than we eat foods like hot dogs or crackers.

- **Variety.** We eat different foods from day to day.

- **Moderation.** We eat only when we're hungry, and we stop when we're full.

Kids can't learn these lessons overnight, but then they don't learn how to walk, how to dress, or how to be polite overnight, either. That's OK. In all of these life arenas, the goal is to help children grow into a more mature way of being. In the case of food, it's to teach children to eventually make healthy choices on their own.

When kids follow the three eating habits, they naturally eat nutritionally. But without these habits, they often eat poorly, even when they're presented with healthy food.

If you're feeling a little skeptical, I don't blame you. It's hard to believe that three little habits could end the food fights and change the way children eat. Believe me, they can. The reason these three habits can work wonders is because they focus directly on teaching your children the eating behaviors you want them to learn. More-

What Kids Hear When You Talk About Food

Kids need a clear and simple basis for understanding healthy eating. Without it, they'll never understand how to make good food decisions because they'll believe that those decisions are mostly arbitrary. If you look at the eating environment through the eyes of a child, you'll see what I mean: One day, parents tell their daughter to eat her veggies because veggies are healthy; another day, the parents tell their daughter she has to eat her veggies because that's what they have cooked; on another day, they tell their daughter she has to eat vegetables if she wants dessert. Sometimes she is supposed to eat three bites; other times she has to eat six. And although her parents are very insistent that she eat vegetables and try new foods at dinnertime, they are content to let her have her favorites at breakfast and lunch.

If the rules about food seem arbitrary, the child thinks those rules can be changed. "If decisions are made because of what my parents want, why can't they be made because of what *I* want?" Most children don't form these thoughts consciously or use words like *arbitrary*, of course, but those are their general sentiments. These unspoken thoughts are also the source of control struggles. In an arbitrary eating environment, eating decisions are up for grabs. How many bites of turkey do I have to eat before I can have a brownie? Let the bidding begin!

And that's why the three habits—proportion, variety, and moderation—are so useful. They offer a clear framework for making your decisions and explaining them to your kids.

over, in contrast to the nutrition mindset, which overloads parents with a ton of details, proportion, variety, and moderation simplify your life. By connecting snacks and meals into a single paradigm, these three habits give you a broader perspective, so that patterns are illuminated, your kids' eating style starts making sense, and fixes become apparent.

In the first part of this book, I describe how well-meaning parents—ones who try really hard to feed their children well—encounter some of the problems and pitfalls that come with the nutrition mindset. The book's second part opens with a method for hitting the reset button on your mindset and for changing the way you interact with your kids when it comes to food. Then you'll learn more about the three habits of proportion, variety, and moderation and how to put them to work in your house. Throughout the chapters, I provide evidence for the teaching approach and also describe the kinds of concrete skills that help kids put the habits into place. These skills include how to:

- Summon the courage to taste something new.

- Snack without ruining dinner.

- Navigate a world filled with tempting (read: *bad*) choices.

- Eat enough at meals—without eating too much.

- Eat something other than their favorite food *every single night*.

Parents come to my workshops or counseling sessions feeling unsure or desperate. They don't yet realize there is a large discrepancy between what they *think* they are teaching their children about eating and what they *are* actually teaching them. Once they begin to close this gap, however, improvement comes swiftly. Although the teaching approach involves commitment and work, parents are amazed by how easy it is to identify the source of their children's food problems and how readily change can be achieved. Parents frequently comment that the information is "revelatory" or "an aha moment." At home, they're more organized and more relaxed at mealtimes. Their picky eaters slowly try and like new foods, the family sits down to the same meal instead of several individually tailored requests, the family eats more food that is wholesome and real, and parents feel that they've found a comfortable middle ground between the extremes of doormat and dictator. These changes take some time, but patience is key to the teaching approach. With this book, I hope to help you resolve your food dilemmas in a way that works.

How Focusing on Nutrition Leads to Poor Habits

One problem with the nutrition mindset is that it doesn't focus on the good habits of proportion, variety, and moderation. But another problem is that it actually leads directly to *bad* eating habits.

How can this be? How can it be true that by worrying so much about calcium, bad fats, protein, and fiber—by devoting so much brain space to remembering which grocery store sells the most palatable whole wheat pizza crust—parents actually teach bad habits?

No parent teaches bad habits on purpose. But there are five traps parents easily fall into when they focus so intently on nutrients. These traps keep parents locked into a cycle that produces, and then reproduces, bad eating habits. In this chapter, I help you see how all that agony over nutrition often leads to overeating, picky eating, junky eating, and all-around stress.

If you see your own tendencies in these traps, know this: Raising kids is hard. Feeding kids is hard, too. What's more, it's almost impossible *not* to fall into these traps. Cut yourself a break.

But realize that whatever it is you're doing now, it's harder than teaching good eating habits. Teaching good eating habits is a lot like teaching your kids to brush their teeth or say please or use the toilet. It takes a lot of repetition, and at first, it's an all-hands-on-deck effort. But once you've got the habit in place, things get much easier. You have to be ready to offer refresher courses, but mostly you will find that your children eat better—and you worry much less about food than you did before. And like all those other lessons you teach your kids, the benefits of healthy eating habits go way beyond the dinner table. Success in this single area of parenting means that *all* the wheels of family life turn more smoothly. There's less stress, anxiety, and conflict; there are more enjoyable times for everyone.

Now let's look at how good parents teach bad habits.

SELECTIVE ATTENTION

Nutrition scientists do fascinating and important work. But nutrition science is a complex field, with thousands of moving parts. For example, the typical food label has around 18 nutrition facts, though some labels list many more. Let's say you serve four foods at each meal, with three meals a day. That's twelve foods multiplied by 18 nutrition facts, which comes to 216 facts to keep track of in one single day. Throw in a couple of snacks and you might need to monitor around 250 food facts or more. And that's assuming you're counting nutrition facts for just one child. Then, if you want to get things exactly right, you'd have to calibrate the nutrients your child actually absorbs because these change according to the combination of foods you're serving and your method of cooking. Let's not even get started on whether organic foods have more nutrients than foods that are conventionally grown. Forget about the fact that nutrition scientists are constantly adding to our knowledge about what's healthful and what's not and that new evidence can cause them to reverse their positions. (The research about eggs has led to so many different conclusions over the years that most people don't even know *what* to think about them anymore. Healthy? Harmful? Anyone?)

Faced with nutrition science overload, most parents I know make an unconscious decision to focus on just a handful of nutrients that seem the most critical either to get into or to keep out of their kids' diets. Their list usually looks like this, though yours might be different:

- Protein

- Calcium

- Fat

- Fiber

- Sugar

- Vitamin C

- Fruits and vegetables

(Never mind that fruits and vegetables aren't nutrients themselves. They're foods that *contain* nutrients. They get a spot on the list anyway, because parents consider them the Holy Grails of healthy eating.)

Let me be clear: I'm not saying that parents really believe that this list encompasses everything they need to know about nutrition science. Most have a sophisticated bank of food information and are familiar with things like antioxidants, omega-3 fatty acids, and the glycemic index, but they draw on the nutrient short list for the majority of their day-to-day decisions.

The nutrient short list is an unconscious way to manage the impossible problem of analyzing a zillion elements of nutrition science and applying them to the kinds of food you shop for and serve. But this solution is a trap that produces some problems of its own. First of all, the focus on nutrients creates a dire sense of emergency. It can make parents think that if their kids don't consume their daily requirement of something on the list, it's just a matter of days before their bones crack or their cells start to shrivel.

Then, as you're casting about for an easy way to get enough calcium or protein into your children, another mental shortcut comes to the rescue: *Selective Attention*. Selective Attention lets you zero in on just a few ingredients of a food—the ingredients you can feel good about—and ignore whatever aspects of the food make you feel bad. Pretty soon, you start making poor food choices, all in the name of nutrition. Do any of the following statements sound familiar?

"He eats a lot of mac 'n' cheese, but at least it's got calcium."

"Nuggets for dinner? At least they've got plenty of protein."

"They get strawberry yogurt tubes for a snack because at least they've got some calcium and fruit."

Of course, parents are aware that these foods aren't *really* good for their kids. (That's why they use the words *at least* a lot.) We know that the presence of one or two nutrients in these foods doesn't neutralize their fatty, sugary, salty punch. But that's what Selective Attention does; it messes with your head. It lets you pretend that the marginally healthy foods your kids prefer are really not that bad for them. It helps you avoid the facts by persuading yourself that if your child's food has one important nutrient, all its bad qualities don't matter. (OK, the bad qualities may still matter to you, but Selective Attention helps you feel better anyway.)

It's not surprising that parents use the Selective Attention approach. Our culture specializes in it. It's how pediatricians and makers of health policy talk, and it's how health information gets communicated. Food manufacturers know this, and they base entire marketing campaigns on appealing to your Selective Attention sensibilities. They take processed foods that are high in sugar, salt, and fat, and they gloss over the bad stuff while trumpeting the presence of one or two nutrients: "Froot Loops is a good source of fiber and made with whole grains," touts the box. Never mind that Froot Loops is also loaded with sugar.

There's another, more insidious, problem with Selective Attention. As the core contributor to the nutrition mindset, Selective Attention distracts parents from the true task at hand. It makes parents think that the big issue is getting certain nutrients into their kids. It's not. The big issue is teaching our children to eat according to the three habits: proportion, variety, and moderation. (Here comes the teaching approach.) We need to shape our kids' behaviors so that it becomes natural for them to eat a wide variety of foods in proportion to their healthy benefits.

This is why Selective Attention is so deadly. *When parents focus on certain nutrients, they often end up serving foods that teach bad habits.* How? By giving parents a sense of nutrition security, Selective Attention prompts parents to feed their children a limited range of inferior foods. A diet like this points kids' taste preferences toward junk and away from all the healthy foods you want them to eat. Think of this as the antiproportion and antivariety diet.

Calcium is a case in point. Sufficient calcium is really not that hard to get: a glass or two of plain milk and some Cheddar cheese are about all that young kids need. (There are other options, too; all plant foods contain at least some calcium. Think kale, tofu, bread.) But to make it easier to get calcium into kids, many schools and parents serve chocolate milk. ("At least it's got calcium!") The strategy works; when kids are given chocolate milk as an option, they ingest more calcium.

But they get a few other things, too. They get sugar: about the same amount (24 grams) as in a Hershey's milk chocolate bar. Some brands of chocolate milk have a little less sugar, true, but some brands have even more. Let your kids drink a bottle of Nesquik chocolate milk and they'll take in 56 grams of sugar.

Moreover, when Selective Attention leads you to use chocolate milk as a way to get some calcium down the hatch, you're not actually teaching kids about healthy eating. You're passing on the Selective Attention point of view, and teaching your children that mixing milk with chocolate somehow negates the sugar, rendering the whole drink healthy (or healthy *enough*). You're also teaching them the *habit* of drinking something highly sweetened.

If you taste a flavor frequently, it becomes the baseline expectation for how food should taste. That's how habits work. Sure, we're all born with preferences for sweet, fatty foods, but if you constantly give your kids sugar (whether it's organic cane sugar, high fructose corn syrup, honey, or any other form of sweetener), you just ramp up that natural preference, making their cravings for sweet things even stronger. Some research suggests that sugar can be addictive, but even if it's not, sweet flavors are certainly habit forming. All flavors are, and so are textures. Regularly give your kids sweet things and they'll expect more sweet things; give them salty and they'll expect more salt; give them fried and they'll want more fried; give them crunchy and they'll want more crunch; give them cheesy and they'll want more cheese.

Worse, the eating habits that are laid down in childhood don't end when childhood is over. Bad eating habits extend themselves into young adulthood. As teens have more freedom to choose from a wider range of foods, they will branch out—not to more healthy foods but to other foods with the same flavor profiles they've come to love. Those foods may have few or no nutrients at all. So when kids who have been raised on chocolate milk are in their teens and twenties, they will naturally reach for something sweet when they are thirsty, and maybe chocolate milk will be their choice. But imagine a sugar-habituated teen, standing in a restaurant and deciding what to drink with lunch. He's going to want something sweet to drink, and given our cultural tendencies, that drink will probably be soda or a sports drink, the kinds of drinks that are a leading cause of obesity. (Did you know that drinking just one 12-ounce sugary beverage a day increases a child's odds of obesity by 60 percent?)

If chocolate milk were the only compromise parents made in the name of nutrition, it might not be such a bad thing. But what happens when parents give their kids chocolate milk for calcium, chicken nuggets for protein, and yogurt tubes for fruit? They may reach their goal of cramming in a few nutrients, but in the process, they will encourage their kids to love foods from the bottom of the nutrition barrel: stuff that's sugary, salty, fatty, or processed. Precisely what most parents want to avoid in the first place!

Plenty of parents ask me how to get their child to like vegetables or plain milk. Believe me, it's possible, and I have lots of ideas for you. But one way to start is by realizing that giving a child chocolate milk, mac 'n' cheese, and nuggets—and all the foods that parents justify through Selective Attention—makes it harder for the child to like the healthy stuff. Kids who regularly eat roasted chicken, for example, usually develop a taste for it. But every chicken nugget makes roasted chicken a harder sell. That's because salty, crunchy chicken nuggets not only train our children's taste buds to want more salty, crunchy chicken nuggets, but also make roasted chicken seem dull and strangely chewy in comparison. The same is true for other foods and flavors. Carrots will never be as satisfyingly crispy as crackers. Even the ripest melons can seem downright tart in comparison to products that have been enhanced with sugar. In comparison to sweetened, fatty, salty, or processed foods, truly wholesome foods will almost always seem less appetizing and less interesting. Naturally healthy foods simply don't taste, look, crunch,

How Parents Unintentionally Shape Eating Habits

When you serve food to your children, you're doing more than providing calories and nutrients. You're also shaping their habits. If you have trouble getting your kids to like healthy food, consider how the types of foods you're serving are shaping your kids' food preferences:

- Sweetened fruit yogurts point kids toward pudding and ice cream.
- Breakfast bars lead to pastries.
- Crackers teach kids to like chips.
- Granola bars aim kids toward cookies.
- Juice sets kids up to drink soda.

The next time you select food for your family, don't ask yourself, Does it have calcium? or Does it have protein? Instead, ask yourself, What *habits* am I teaching?

swoosh, or swirl the same as kid-friendly foods do. So if your child is rejecting plain milk and other healthy foods, like fresh produce, the habit of consuming a diet filled with foods that are amped up to please your child's taste buds might just be to blame.

HEALTHIFIED FOODS

Nutrition traps can be hard for even the most alert parent to spot. Parents come to me all the time for help with picky eating, food refusal, and other problems, saying, "I can't figure out what the problem is. I serve only healthy foods!" And they're right; most of the foods these parents serve seem pretty healthy. But the parents are caught in a trap nevertheless, and this trap is the reason their kids aren't eating as well as they'd like. I'm speaking of the tendency to take junky or mediocre foods and "healthify" them.

EXAMPLES OF HEALTHIFIED FOODS

- Chips made with vegetables

- Pizza made with whole wheat crust

- Muffins made with healthy add-ins

- Mac 'n' cheese spiked with cauliflower

- Brownies baked with black bean puree

If you think about food solely in terms of nutrients—if you have a nutrition mindset—the healthifying strategy makes a lot of sense. It solves a problem for you. If your child wants to eat muffins for breakfast every morning, but you're concerned about the refined flour and sugar that are in most muffins, you can stay up late and make your own from whole grains. You can leave out the white sugar and sweeten the batter with apple juice. Toss in a handful of flax seeds for fiber and add some blueberries. It's midnight and you're exhausted, but at least you've got a muffin that is much healthier. Right?

Well, yes. But what kinds of habits are you teaching?

If you offer your child healthified muffins every morning, you are teaching your child:

- It's OK to eat the same food every day, or nearly every day.

- Breakfast is a time to eat fluffy, sweet foods.

- To prefer the taste and texture of baked goods rather than of fresh foods.

These lessons don't teach your child healthy habits. They don't teach her how to manage the experience of new foods, how to develop an appreciation for other kinds of breakfast foods, like eggs or cereal, or how to incorporate variety into her diet. What these lessons *do* teach is how to become a rigid eater. A muffin-head! And consider this: Not every muffin your muffin-head eats will be the healthy kind, especially when she's older and looking over the options (like blueberry strudel, chocolate chip, and cinnamon crumb cake) on a breakfast cart.

The desire to make "bad" food "good" is natural. One time, a mother participating in one of my seminars told me she thought the solution to the problem of cream cheese—it has too much saturated fat and not enough calcium to make it into the USDA's Dairy Group—was to fortify it, not to change her kids' eating habits. I understand where this mother was coming from, but her logic was off. Turning harmful foods into healthy ones is a false win that ultimately makes your life harder—because healthified foods train your child's taste buds to resist foods that are naturally fresh and good for them.

Consider what happened to Lana. When I met her, Lana was giving her two sons pizza for dinner almost every night. Lana felt bad about all the pizza, but she felt good knowing that the pizza she served was made with a whole wheat crust. Her boys liked it, and Lana wasn't sure what else to do. She had trouble getting her sons to eat other foods as easily, and she was tired of the food fights.

And there's the trap. Lana began serving pizzas because her sons complained about eating other foods. By healthifying the crust, Lana had convinced herself that it was OK to feed her sons pizza every day. This strategy worked to keep the peace, and there's a lot to be said for peace at the dinner table. But now that her kids were used to eating pizza all the time, their minds and their mouths expected pizza every night. When they looked at their pizza, her sons learned something: This is what dinner is. This is what it tastes like.

When Lana thought about dinner from a nutrition perspective, all she saw were the whole grains in the crust. That made her pies a big improvement on the ones sold at the local pizzeria. But when Lana saw dinner from a habits perspective, she could see that the tastes, texture, and entire experience of eating her healthified pizza was a long way from the foods she hoped her sons would eat—things like chicken teriyaki, beans and rice, broccoli, and someday even salad—and that each pizza she served was pushing her kids toward more pizza.

Of course, change wasn't easy. There's no magic bullet. But by switching up what she served a little more frequently, Lana was able to start shifting how her children ate. More importantly, Lana finally saw the *big* picture. She learned that healthified food is an ingenious sleight of hand that encourages parents to fix their attention narrowly on a single food and to overlook their children's overall pattern—or habit—of eating.

THE NUTRITION ZONE

Some parents designate breakfast, lunch, and dinner as *Nutrition Zones*, the times when healthy food is served.

Having healthy meals is great. But what about the rest of the day? What about snacks?

I'm not saying all snacks have to be good for you; what a boring world that would be.

But it's easy to slip into the idea that snacks stand firmly outside the Nutrition Zone and that snacks *always* have a free pass to be junky or mediocre.

Parents don't start out thinking about snacks this way. Indeed, when our children are infants, we are pretty comfortable serving mini-meals all day long. We give our small children nutritious food, such as oatmeal or fruit and vegetable purees, scattered throughout the day.

As our children grow older, though, we are inclined to make more a of a distinction between meals and snacks. Snack time becomes a time for prepackaged snack foods like pretzels or crackers, which are primarily stomach fillers with little or no nutritional value. Or snack time becomes a time for candy, potato chips, cookies, or ice cream. It's like setting aside time each day as extra-calorie time or high-fat time or cavity time.

What's interesting is that parents whose children have eaten well at mealtimes are more likely to indulge their kids with extras. It may seem that junk is less damaging when it "complements" a healthy diet, but really, junk is junk. It's not like candy and chips are any healthier for kids who have eaten their veggies. (It's sad, but broccoli does not inoculate kids against sugar!)

The junk quality of most snacks aside, kids add a *lot* of calories with snacks. Children now consume more than 27 percent of their daily calories from snacks. On average, children consume just under 600 daily calories—slightly more than the number of calories in a McDonald's Big Mac—between meals. High-calorie snacking is one reason so many adults are overweight. Are you sure that you want to train your children in this habit?

All those calories from snacks can have two effects:

- They fill up kids' tummies so that they're not hungry for meals. If meals are when you serve the healthy stuff, that's a problem. It forces you to make a choice: Are you going to demand that your child eat when she's not hungry, or are you going to let her skip the meal and then fill up on more empty calories at the next snack?

- They dull your child's sense of satiety and lead to stronger cravings for even more snacks. Manufacturers have found the "bliss point" at which snacks are made the most desirable. High-calorie snacks, particular those high in sugar, salt, and fat, stimulate our appetites for more snacks. They set in motion a cycle of desire and consumption, so kids (and adults) keep eating.

The Nutrition Zone is one of the ways parents respond to nutrition information overload, and it can feel like a lifesaver. By limiting the number of times each day parents have to think about nutrition, it also limits the number of times they have to (potentially) fight with their kids about food. But that's the trap. Subpar snacking actually makes your life worse. Not only does it spiral your kids' tastes downward, so that they crave a bigger and bigger proportion of junk, but it also makes mealtimes matter more than they should. They become the *only* chances you've got to serve the good-for-you stuff.

Dinner, the big daddy of the day, bears the brunt of our nutrition goals. That's why almost every family I know obsesses about dinner. "How can I get my son to eat a better dinner?" "How can I get my son to eat more at dinner?" "How can I get my son to eat vegetables at dinner?"

The answer, ironically, is to think about snacks. That's what I told Anita. Anita made sure to serve her three children one vegetable, once a day, at dinner. Dinner was always miserable. The kids would see the vegetables on their plates and complain. Anita would scold and cajole them, and tell the kids to eat half of whatever amount was left on their plates. Usually a few more vegetables got eaten, but not many.

I understood Anita's logic: "It's a nightly battle to get my kids to eat just one serving of vegetables. If I serve vegetables more than once a day, I'm committing myself to a lot of fighting."

It doesn't work that way, though. Kids reject vegetables when they're not used to them. If Anita's kids had more exposure to vegetables at snack times (and at other meals), they would be more willing to eat them at dinner. It may sound like circular logic, but it's true. If you want your kids to eat more vegetables, they've got to become more familiar with vegetables.

I'm not suggesting that Anita should start serving salads for breakfast, although she could, and families in other cultures do, but there are lots of ways to squeeze more veggies into the day. How about topping toast with cream cheese and cherry tomatoes (or cucumbers, or avocado, or all three) for breakfast? Dipping carrot sticks into guacamole for snack? And serving vegetable spring rolls or vegetable soup for lunch? Every bite adds up. More importantly, every bite gets kids more comfortable with the way vegetables look, taste, and smell. Then, when dinnertime rolls around, vegetables seem like a go-to food, not a side dish to fight over and resist.

There's another way in which serving vegetables throughout the day would encourage Anita's kids to eat more of them at dinner. If Anita knew by dinnertime that her kids had gotten in *even a couple* of carrots or grape tomatoes, she wouldn't care as much about what (or how much) her kids ate at dinner. That would allow her to take some of the pressure off regarding dinner vegetables—and that's a good thing. Without the pressure to eat vegetables, Anita's kids would probably eat more of them.

However, because Anita thought of meals as the Nutrition Zone, she was trapped into a cycle that is hard to break: Dinner is a struggle; parents worry that their kids are hungry, so they give them snacks they enjoy; because the snacks that kids enjoy are nutritionally inferior, parents worry more about dinner; that worry makes parents bribe, beg, barter, and coax their kids into eating a few more bites; kids respond negatively to the pressure; and the cycle starts all over again.

Now, I'm definitely *not* saying that every bite has to be nutritious. There has to be a place for sweets and treats in all of our diets.

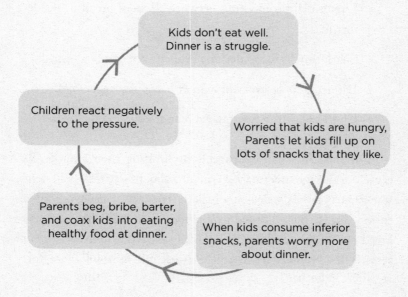

(You won't find me giving up chocolate chip cookies anytime soon.) But the Nutrition Zone mentality has got to go because it produces a cycle of pressure and despair. Bottom line: Break out of the Nutrition Zone and you are more likely to spread healthy food throughout the day, to intersperse treats when the time is right—in other words, to produce a proportionally correct diet and to teach your kids to be more open to enjoying the healthy stuff. Stay within it, and you're doomed.

FALSE CHOICES

There's an industry working overtime to convince parents that there are certain foods that you have to serve in certain circumstances. Here are some of the food groupings as we've come to know them:

- Breakfast is for bready products, eggs, and cereal.

- Lunch is for something between slices of bread or inside a tortilla.

- Snack time is for something crunchy out of a box or bag.

- Dinner is for a savory protein or pasta plus vegetables.

- Children are supposed to eat bland, kid-friendly foods.

This thinking restricts parents by limiting their choices. Because the average supermarket contains about forty thousand items, sometimes parents welcome a little restriction. It makes shopping easier. But if you're limited by the idea that lunch has to feature bread or tortillas, and if you combine that with the constraints of serving kid-friendly food, you've ruled out most of those forty thousand items before you even walk in the door. They're literally off the table! Even if some of those foods are delicious. Even if you would serve them if it were evening instead of afternoon. Even if they're your child's favorite color. And even if it's a food like miso soup, which Americans don't think of as kid friendly but is eaten for breakfast by many of the seventeen million children in Japan.

Another problem is that when you serve predictable kinds of foods at predictable times, you're creating a limited sensory experience. Even if you serve Goldfish crackers for a snack one day, pretzels the next day, and graham crackers the day after that, your kids are getting used to a similar texture: crispy. The same goes for sandwiches. Kids who eat the same kinds of things at the same time of day, over and over, are more likely to become rigid in their approach to food—and rigidity is the opposite of being willing to try new things.

I tell parents that the easiest and fastest way they can add variety to their children's diets is by expanding their idea of *when* their kids eat *what*. Everyone enjoys breakfast for dinner, but you don't have to stop there. You can serve falafel for breakfast or chicken soup for a snack. If pasta, hot dogs, and chicken nuggets are an acceptable option in your home for dinner, they're also OK at other times. (And if you wouldn't serve Goldfish crackers at breakfast, maybe you should reconsider whether they're suitable for so many snacks.)

I know that mixing up meals this way doesn't seem as though it will get you very far toward the goal of increasing the amount of variety in your child's diet, but it will—and not just because it will automatically add dozens of dishes to the menu. Breaking out of the trap of False Choices will also change the kinds of foods your kids *expect* to eat at any given meal. It's only when their expectations change that kids' food choices can also change.

The worst problem with False Choices, though, isn't that they discourage variety, though that's bad enough. The worst problem is that they discourage variety *and* lure parents into serving inferior foods to their kids. When you feel restricted to only a handful of "legal" foods to serve in a particular circumstance, you start making your decisions based on the relative health merits of foods in the category. Often this means pitting one bad choice against another.

This is why parents end up saying things like

"I give Sally bagels for breakfast because they're not as sweet as muffins."

"Justin gets crackers after school because they're healthier than potato chips."

"I make buttered noodles for dinner because they're better than McDonald's."

See the False Choice? The question isn't whether buttered noodles are healthier than McDonald's, or whether crackers are better than chips. The real question is, Are any of these foods healthy? Often, the answer is no.

It can be kind of shocking to step back from the trap of False Choices and look at some popular food items through a different lens. For example, many of us serve bagels because they seem better for our kids than other breakfast foods, such as doughnuts and sweet muffins. Actually, an even better choice than a bagel would be . . . a slice of cake. A plain bagel with cream cheese from a place like Panera Bread has 480 calories and 20 grams of fat. One slice of Entenmann's chocolate fudge cake has 200 fewer calories, and about half the fat. The cake even has the same amount of fiber! Throw in a glass of milk and you're good to go. Most of us would feel a little weird serving cake for breakfast—though on occasion it would be a fun thing to do. But the magic of False Choices has us believing that cake is a health disaster, while bagels are somehow pretty good for you.

Once again, I'm not saying there isn't room in your child's diet for crackers or that you have to ban all bagels, or even McDonald's. I'm saying something more radical: You need to break out of the trap of False Choices because it dials down your expectations for what constitutes an acceptable diet. When you make the best choice from the mediocre middle, you end up stuck in the mediocre middle. And when you limit the range of choices you give your kids, you reinforce their narrow palates rather than expand them.

EAT SOME MORE

So far, all the nutrition traps I've talked about get kids stuck in either picky eating or eating too many foods that aren't very good for them. This last nutrition habit, Eat Some More, leads to a different bad habit: eating too much food.

Ironically, parents are lured into the Eat Some More trap when they serve foods they think of as healthy. When the good stuff is on the table, parents, shall we say, *encourage* their kids to eat more than they normally would:

"Eat two more bites."

"If you want a brownie, you've got to eat your broccoli."

"No TV tonight until you've eaten all your dinner."

Eat Some More is kind of like nutrition insurance. In pursuit of nutrition goals that they can't quite pinpoint, the parents I know are never quite satisfied that their children have consumed enough calcium, enough protein, or even enough calories. Most parents settle for a simple solution: feed more. In this way, Eat Some More is another simplification strategy that parents use to cope with nutrition information overload, thinking, "I don't really know how much protein you need or how much you've already eaten. Just to be safe, eat some more." Eat Some More also solves the practical problem of getting kids to eat enough at meals so they don't have a hunger-driven temper tantrum later or beg for a snack just before bedtime. It's easy to see why one team of researchers recently concluded that getting kids to eat more at meals was the overriding goal of the majority of parents of young children.

Like all the traps, Eat Some More is counterproductive to your goal of getting your kids to eat well. Pressuring kids to eat more at a meal can sometimes make them eat less (it's a control thing). Even if you do get your kids to consume a few more mouthfuls of dinner, what have you really achieved? Most of the time, those "two more bites" are not enough food to prevent a major hunger meltdown, not enough to forestall a future snack attack, and certainly not a huge improvement in terms of nutrition. The only thing you've gained is a temporary win, followed by more struggle. In the process, you've taught your kids a slew of bad eating habits.

Here's how it happens. Let's say your children are less than enthusiastic about eating vegetables. You decide to make vegetable eating a condition for getting dessert. (I call this the Dessert Deal.) Chances are good that your strategy will work. Most kids will do just about anything to get to the goodies, even if it means they have to choke down a few more of those (in their opinion, abominable) peas you insist on serving. They eat the peas; you serve up the pie. Everybody wins. Think beyond the immediate meal, however, and the picture doesn't look so rosy.

For starters, the Dessert Deal doesn't actually teach kids to like peas. If it did, you'd do this a few times and then your kids would start eating veggies on their own. You wouldn't have to negotiate *every single night*. Instead, the Dessert Deal teaches kids that dessert is really desirable (after all, if dessert is the reward, it's got to be good) and that vegetables are a disgusting chore. Otherwise, you wouldn't need a reward for eating them. The lesson that peas aren't tasty is one that lasts a lifetime. One study of college students in Texas found that 72 percent of the students who had been forced to eat a particular food as a child wouldn't willingly eat that food today.

There's a bigger problem with the Eat Some More strategy. Pressuring kids to eat more food teaches kids . . . to eat more food, regardless of how hungry they are. Kids' thoughts then run something like this: "I was kind of full. Mom made me eat a few more bites to get dessert. Then I was really full. I still wanted my dessert, though. Now I'm stuffed." I'm pretty sure that eating-until-stuffed isn't quite the habit you are hoping to establish.

Over time, the news gets even grimmer. When pressured to eat more than they normally would, kids, even very young ones, learn to disregard their own internal eating instincts. Instead of looking inward to assess how hungry or full they are, kids start looking to external cues to help them decide when, and how much, to eat. That puts kids at risk of becoming overeaters, and not just in the short run, either. When we spend the first few years of our children's lives pushing them to eat more, we shouldn't be surprised when they have to spend the rest of their lives trying to eat less. Habits earned early in life tend to stick around.

"Just a few more bites" is only one way kids learn to overeat. Here's another way: Many parents plop huge portions onto their child's plates, knowing full well that they've just served up significantly more than their child will ever eat. Parents do this because they know that people generally eat more when they're served more, and parents have done the math: "My child usually eats one-fourth of what I serve. If I serve a bigger portion, the one-fourth that she eats will be bigger, too."

Unfortunately, increasing portion size is another one of those short-term solutions that produces its own long-term problems. Kids who get used to eating a lot start to think of *a lot* as normal. It becomes their *consumption norm*, the amount they strive to replicate each and every time they eat. Even when what they're eating is healthy, they still learn to eat too much.

I know it feels as if your children would never touch a vegetable if you stopped pressuring them. However, if I had to choose between teaching my daughter to eat vegetables and teaching her not to overeat, I would choose the latter. (Fortunately, I'm going to show you how to achieve both.) You can't ignore the statistics. More than one-third of all American children are overweight or obese— not just because of what our kids are eating but because of *how much* we're teaching them to eat as well.

DON'T DITCH NUTRITION, JUST THE NUTRITION MINDSET

It's a frustrating paradox of modern parenting that if you focus on nutrition, your kids will most likely develop bad eating habits. If you focus on teaching the habits you want them to have, however, the nutrition will naturally fall into place. That's because habits reflect behavior; nutrition reflects food.

You can do a lot to help your children learn healthy eating habits by ditching the nutrition mindset, but you don't have to ditch nutrition entirely. Simply dial down some of the noise. In her book *What to Eat*, the noted nutritionist Marion Nestle writes, "The basic principles of good diets are so simple that I can summarize them in just ten words: eat less, move more, eat lots of fruits and vegetables. For additional clarification, a five-word modifier helps: Go easy on junk foods." And, I would add: Think about long-term habits.

To escape the nutrition traps, you need a whole new way of thinking. The teaching approach is about much more than providing food; it's really about your parenting, too. As the next chapter discusses, if you want to change the way your children eat, what you have to do is change the way you interact with your kids around food.

If You Had *My* Kid, You'd Understand

How Your Issues Hold You Hostage

We've talked about the thoughts and behaviors that lure you into the nutrition traps; now it's time to look even more deeply. If your child has acquired a handful of challenging habits, then chances are you probably have a couple hanging around in your closet, too. I'm not talking about your eating habits, though. I'm talking about your parenting habits. Those struggles you have getting your kids to eat right? I hate to be the one to break it to you, but sometimes you are your own worst enemy. Every struggling parent describes something—an unwillingness to let her child experience any amount of hunger, the belief that kids have a free pass to enjoy fun foods that are unhealthy for adults, the desire to avoid conflict—that competes with her efforts to teach her children how to eat well.

In fact, we *all* have times when something gets in the way of teaching healthy eating habits. Years ago, I was traveling to Australia with my then-sixteen-month-old daughter. I'd known since her birth that I wanted to feed my child well, but on that particular day

I *also* knew that I didn't want her to spend the flight crying or being uncomfortable when the air pressure changed during takeoff.

So I used a steady stream of Goldfish crackers (a snack she considered a rare treat) to keep my daughter occupied and quiet while other passengers were boarding the plane. Then I used a full bottle of milk to keep her ears from hurting during takeoff. What followed wasn't pretty. Let's just say that thirty minutes into a thirty-hour journey my little darling lost her lunch. Onto my lap. And I learned my lesson: Pay attention to why (and how much) you feed your kids. I should have entertained my daughter during boarding without food. Then I wouldn't have overfed her. I also wouldn't have risked teaching her to use food for the wrong reasons.

Feeding kids is a juggling act. One minute we're throwing one ball into the air—*teaching kids to eat right*—and the next we're tossing up another ball—*keeping kids quiet*. Of course, if you know anything about juggling, you know how easy it is to drop a ball. And that's what I had done on the plane: I had dropped *teaching kids to eat right* and, instead, had put my effort into tossing around *buy some time*, *give my daughter a treat*, and *ward off takeoff trauma*. You see where that got me.

In sociology, we call this kind of situation a conflict between your manifest and latent goals. Your manifest goal—in this case teaching kids to eat right—is your conscious motivation. In contrast, latent goals often go unspoken. A dad who gives his son pizza for dinner when the rest of the family is having fish may have the latent goal of avoiding a conflict over food. A mom who lets her kid eat a sleeve of Girl Scout cookies before dinner may have the latent goal of having some peace and quiet after a long day.

These unspoken goals are really powerful because they're driven by your emotions and by your fears, your hopes, and the way you show your love. If you find it incredibly difficult to feed your child the way you want to, it may be because your emotions have, in a sneaky way, taken over.

This is what happened to Audrey. Audrey wanted her daughter, Nia, to eat well, but she also worried that Nia wouldn't eat *enough*. A lot of parents worry about their children's weight, and often with good reason. In Audrey's case, her daughter had been small at birth and didn't eat very well in her first few months. Having an underweight baby can be scary, especially for a first-time parent, and the experience left Audrey terrified that her daughter might always be a little undernourished or not grow properly. But Nia was now three years old and in the seventy-fifth percentile for weight; her pediatrician was happy with her growth. Audrey, however, couldn't let go of her determination to get more food into Nia.

Like most toddlers, Nia made her food preferences very clear. At meals she would push her plate away and demand one of her favorite foods as a replacement. Audrey, always fearful that her daughter might not eat enough, succumbed. This solution of giving Nia whatever she wanted started out fine. Nia ate just enough strawberries and apples to make Audrey feel good. But this solution created its own problem. Over time, the list of foods Nia was willing to eat became shorter and shorter. That's what kids do when they are using food as an arena for control—they become more and more controlling. By the time Audrey called me, her daughter would eat only four kinds of foods: pizza, cream cheese on bread, baked beans, and yogurt.

Nia's pediatrician had recommended that Audrey take a tough line with the toddler. "Tell her to either eat what's on her plate or go to bed hungry," he said. This strategy works for some parents, but it would never work for Audrey because it would trigger her fears far too much. That's why Audrey had never even tried it. Instead, I encouraged Audrey to talk about her fears and about why she was still so concerned about Nia's growth. I then helped Audrey see that her goal of giving Nia healthy meals was in conflict with her goal of getting food into Nia at any cost. Until that changed, Nia's diet was going to stay the same.

Every single one of us will sometimes use food in a way that conflicts with the bigger goal of teaching kids to eat well. There are seven common categories parents generally fall into when hung up by their inner issues. As you read through the parenting types described in this chapter, don't be surprised if you find yourself represented in several categories. Don't worry. We all dip in and out of issues as they become more or less pertinent to our lives. Hang-ups that are merely temporary or low level are good to recognize, but they don't define how you feed your children. They're like moderate-force winds: You feel their effects, but they won't blow you totally off course.

On the other hand, you will probably read about one or two issues that really seem to resonate. Pay attention. These are the hang-ups that are most likely to undermine your feeding efforts.

Also, don't think you have to completely fix your issues to teach your kids to eat right. You don't, at least not right away. At this point you simply need to understand how your hang-ups affect the way you feed your kids. That way, your latent goals will have much less power over you. That alone can be life changing.

HUNGER AVOIDERS

Hunger Avoiders fear their kids feeling even the itsy-bitsiest hunger. You know you're a Hunger Avoider if you do one of the following when your child refuses food that you've provided:

You immediately offer your child a substitute that you know he'll eat.

You beg, plead, cajole, and threaten your child, and then offer him a substitute that you know he'll eat.

You never encounter this situation because you automatically provide your child a meal you know he'll eat.

Parents become Hunger Avoiders for lots of reasons. Some people, like Audrey, end up there because they worry about their children being underweight. Other parents are susceptible to being Hunger Avoiders because they become concerned about food consumption at certain times of the day. Breakfast, for instance, can be a tremendous trigger. This is Dana's issue. She worries about sending her son off to school if he hasn't eaten enough breakfast. As a result, she finds herself constantly caving in to Hayden's demands for pancakes, waffles, and muffins, when she would rather he ate eggs, yogurt, and cereal. On the other hand, Dana isn't a Hunger Avoider in the evening. Then, she's entirely comfortable letting Hayden go to bed even if he has completely refused to eat his dinner.

Lots of parents, though, are Hunger Avoiders all the time, usually because their little eaters have convinced them that they'd rather starve than eat something they think is yucky or not exactly what they want at that precise moment. I sympathize. It is really difficult to set boundaries around food when you're worried that your children are going to die of hunger. In fact, I'd say it's practically impossible. That's how Hunger Avoiders end up feeding to their kids' taste preferences. They fear that their children will refuse meals—and therefore starve themselves—unless they are served their favorite foods. This fear leads parents to provide a monotonous, unvaried diet, with the same three or four foods trotted out over and over again.

Hunger Avoiders also tend to raise kids who are big snackers, thinking, "He was starving. How could I say no to a couple of crackers?" A couple of crackers may seem like no big deal. But look at the pattern you're establishing and you'll see a different picture. Children who can snack whenever they want to have no reason to eat at mealtimes. In this way, ever-present snacks feed the fight.

Hunger Avoiders have kids who know that *their* hunger is *your* issue, and they use this power to get what they want. Linda and Kurt found this out the hard way when their son, Sam, a headstrong four-year-old with low weight and a small appetite, ruled the roost with his hunger demands. Sam got milk whenever he wanted milk, cookies whenever he wanted cookies, and his parents' attention whenever he said, "I'm hungry." It didn't matter that one of Sam's favorite foods, milk, is healthy. What mattered is that Sam was using repeated requests for milk as a way to control his parents.

Linda and Kurt didn't mind Sam's demands too much during the day. It meant that Sam might actually eat without a struggle. The problem was that Sam had taken to waking his parents up early, five or six o'clock in the morning, with screams that he was starving. Linda and Kurt would reluctantly get up to make breakfast, and then Sam would simply pick at it.

Of course, it turned out that Sam wasn't really starving. In fact, he was hardly even hungry at all. Here's how we discovered the truth. I advised Linda and Kurt to tell Sam that they would put a bowl of dry cereal on the coffee table each night so that it would be waiting there for him the moment he got up. They also told Sam that when he was done eating he should play with his toys until they awoke. The first morning Sam ate the cereal and then began to play. After that, however, Sam typically skipped the cereal, but he would play quietly by himself until his parents got out of bed.

It would be nice to think that the cereal solution worked because it beat Sam at his own game, but that wasn't really the secret to

Linda and Kurt's success. Addressing *their* fears was the key. Knowing that Sam had easy access to food reassured Linda and Kurt that Sam would be able to eat if he genuinely wanted to, and that gave them the freedom to set firmer boundaries, and to sleep a little bit later in the morning—sometimes even past 7:00.

Linda and Kurt had unintentionally taught Sam that if he acted hungry, he could get his parents to jump. But that wasn't the only lesson Linda and Kurt were inadvertently teaching. By doing anything to keep him from being hungry, they were also demonstrating to Sam that hunger is a feeling to avoid. That's a problem, because an inability to tolerate even a little bit of hunger is a well-known precursor to overeating. (Overeating might not concern you today, but it will down the road, when your kids are at an age when they have more access to food and are more vulnerable to weight gain. Avoiding hunger is a hard habit to break.)

Here's an important truth for Hunger Avoiders to hear: It's impossible for parents to know how much food their kids need to eat. True, there are guidelines, but because you never really know how much energy your children are burning up or how fast they're growing, you can't ever be sure how much food they really need to eat at any given moment. In the end, the only way to be sure that your kids are eating the right amount is to teach them to be their own eating experts. I'll describe this in more detail in Chapter 8.

PEACEMAKERS

You're probably a Peacemaker if you think, "I'm going to make chicken for dinner, but Jane won't eat it without a fuss, and getting into a struggle tonight simply isn't worth the hassle. I'll give her microwave mac 'n' cheese instead."

You're almost certainly a Peacemaker if, after Jane turns her nose up at the macaroni and cheese, you pour her a bowl of her favorite cereal instead.

And you're definitely a Peacemaker if you then dump the cereal down the drain when Jane starts to complain, "I changed my mind. I don't want this kind of cereal after all."

On the surface, Peacemakers resemble Hunger Avoiders. Many Hunger Avoiders would also have let Jane skip the chicken, the macaroni, and the cereal. Here's the difference: Hunger Avoiders give in to their children's demands to ensure that they eat. Peacemakers give in to their children's demands to avoid conflict.

- You're a Hunger Avoider if you'd rather give your child Pop-Tarts than let her go hungry, even though Pop-Tarts make you cringe.

- You're a Peacemaker if you'd rather give your child Pop-Tarts than let her be unhappy, even though Pop-Tarts make you cringe.

I'm not saying that every parent who cuts a deal with her kid is a chronic Peacemaker. There are definitely times when a peacemaking approach is called for. For years, I routinely gave in to my young daughter's demands to wear her winter coat backward—yes, zipped up the back, kind of like a straightjacket—but that doesn't make me a Peacemaker. (I even used to let her pull her hood up over her face. She had a hoot as I steered her down the street.) In this instance, indulging my daughter was an easy way to get the job done. Coat on. Child warm. What more can you ask for?

Most parents occasionally bend and bargain to skirt a conflict. Peacemakers go further, though. Peacemakers routinely go out of their way to avoid causing their kids any kind of distress. They have trouble setting limits; they give their children unhealthy foods, saying, "But he likes it!" Peacemakers feel as if it borders on abuse to serve foods their children don't really love, even though those parents know their kids need to be exposed to different foods to expand their palates. Peacemakers also let their children eat pretty much when and how much they want, even when what they're really thinking is, "That snack will definitely ruin your dinner, young lady."

Meredith is a classic Peacemaker. Her son, Alex, steadfastly refuses to eat anything other than a handful of favorites. Although Meredith wishes her five-year-old would eat a broader range of foods, she doesn't like upsetting him. Partly this is because Meredith wants Alex to be happy, and partly it's because she doesn't like creating tension with anyone. When I first met Meredith, I encouraged her to implement what I call the Rotation Rule. It's an easy technique that would get Alex used to the *idea* of eating different foods on different days—an important first step in broadening his palate—without asking him to actually eat anything new. With the Rotation Rule, Alex could eat any of his favorites for dinner—chicken nuggets, hot dogs, pizza—with one restriction: He couldn't eat the same food two nights in a row. (I'll discuss the Rotation Rule in more depth in the next chapter.)

Although Meredith agreed with the Rotation Rule in principle, she had trouble putting it into practice. On the first night, Alex chose pizza for dinner, and Meredith happily fixed it for him. On the second night, however, Alex again chose pizza. Instead of insisting that Alex pick something else from his list of favorites, Meredith gave in to his demands.

Peacemakers often worry that setting limits is disrespectful. They prefer to nudge and negotiate instead: "Don't you think it would be nice to have a hot dog tonight? Remember we talked about eating something different tonight because you had pizza last night. No? You want pizza? OK."

This strategy only makes matters worse. By asking kids to make a change and then giving in when they refuse, you inadvertently teach them to become even more obstinate. Although you may think that it's kinder not to impose your will on your kids, that it's better to appeal to their logic, it's not. When it comes to eating, kids like Alex aren't operating from a thought-out, reasonable position. They're going with their gut (quite literally) and operating from an emotional and irrational space. Researchers who study brain development tell us that when children are being driven by emotion, trying to use logic will always be a losing approach. It's much more effective to help kids change by mapping out a plan of limits and choices, with small, doable steps. In the next chapter, we'll start talking about ways to do that.

IT'S-JUST-A-PHASERS

When it comes to child development, It's-Just-a-Phasers know their stuff. They know that infants are born with a preference for sweet foods, that toddlers go through a phase of throwing food from their high chairs, and that two-year-olds have a period during which they reject new foods. (If you know that this last stage is called the "neophobic phase," I'm impressed. You really do know your stuff.)

It's-Just-a-Phasers—let's call them IJPs—are great at empathizing with their young children's struggles to develop and grow. The problem with IJPs is that they think there's no choice but to wait out whatever phase their kids are in. Are the kids throwing food? Pleading nonstop for pasta? Insisting that they will eat eggs *only* if they're the eggs that Daddy makes? "Oh, well," say the IJPs, "this behavior is developmentally appropriate. There's nothing we can do but give in. One day they'll grow out of it."

It's easy to see how people become IJPs. Everywhere you look, parents are inundated with information about their children's stages of development. I'm not knocking this. When your kid acts like a little monster, it helps you take it less personally when you know that it's *normal* for him to act, well, like a little monster at this point in his development. The problem is that if you've read the usual food advice—which amounts to "Keep trying, but don't expect too much from your children when they're in a phase"—it's tempting to think there's nothing you can do about how your child eats. Indeed, from this perspective, your only choice is to ride it out. Or, if you have a food thrower, get a dog.

Waiting it out doesn't really work, though, because it's unclear what you're waiting for—perhaps a developmental stage when kids naturally love sautéed kale? A phase when they suddenly stop liking sugar? While you're waiting for those stages to arrive, your kids' unhealthy eating habits are solidifying, increasing the chances that those stages will *never* come.

If you're an IJP, here's the cure: Instead of seeing your child's developmental stage as a roadblock, think of it as a teaching moment. I often ask parents to imagine that their child is experiencing a period of separation anxiety, a normal phase of development that strikes children around the same time that many toddlers also become less adventurous eaters. In the case of separation anxiety, would you say, "Oh well, I guess I can't leave my child's side until this stage is over?" I bet not. Instead, you'd probably say, "This phase is going to be hard for her; how can I help her learn to cope when I'm away?" You can do the same with food by saying to yourself, "This is the phase where my kid throws his sippy cup. I can appreciate that this is normal, but I can also teach him that mealtimes aren't the time for throwing things."

I'm thinking here of my client Sandy, whose son, Luke, was extraordinarily shy during his preschool years. He was afraid of anything new, whether it was new people or new foods. When it

If You Had *My* Spouse, You'd Understand

One woman said to me, "My husband loves potato chips and gives them to the kids all the time. When I tell them not to eat the chips, I feel like I'm getting in between my spouse and my children."

She has a point. You don't want to turn your children's food choices into a judgment against their other parent. And a stressful eating environment, with parents fighting over what their children should eat, is even worse for kids than unhealthy foods.

If you have a similar situation at home, you and your spouse must come to an agreement about how you're going to feed the kids. You may have to relax your standards a little to find a middle ground. In one family, the father was very overweight and didn't want any limits on how much or what his son could eat. The mother, who was afraid the child would become overweight too, wanted very clear limits. They found a middle ground by agreeing that there would be times (such as family picnics) when Dad could decide the menu—anything would go. In return, he would support Mom on the menus she planned for every day. Both parents agreed not to fight about food in front of their son.

Another way to handle this situation is to lay down rules for your children but let them know that adults have the power to make their own decisions. You can say, "Dad can snack whenever he wants to. When you're older, you can, too. But for now, you can have just one snack in the afternoon."

came to social situations, Sandy's response was spot on. Instead of keeping Luke at home—as he preferred—she was careful to expose him to a steady stream of playdates, enrichment classes, and group activities. Sandy was understanding of Luke's resistance, but she was also firm: "I knew I had to keep exposing Luke to different people to make him more comfortable. If I didn't, new social situations were only going to get harder and harder for him. I did my best to smooth the way for Luke, but I never backed down." This is the teaching approach at its most loving.

It never occurred to Sandy that she could do the same thing with Luke's fear of new foods. Instead, she fed him a repetitive diet of safe and easy foods that he felt comfortable with. As a consequence, Luke's ease with people evolved, while his eating became more rigid. But when Sandy realized that she could teach Luke to approach new foods in the same way she taught him to approach new people, things got much better. Later in the book, I offer some effective ways to introduce kids to new food.

I'm not saying that children don't bring their (sometimes difficult) personalities and stages of development into the feeding dynamic. They do, and parents have the job of understanding their child's temperament and level of maturity. But when parents *completely* cater to their kids' culinary demands, they end up reinforcing their children's pickiness rather than taking steps to eradicate it. The longer you wait to teach your children good habits, the harder it will be for them to learn them.

NUTRITIONISTAS

Nutritionistas have stressful lives. They're so worried about getting nutrients into their children that they're always on the lookout for how much protein, calcium, and fiber their kids have eaten that day.

If you are a Nutritionista, a partial day in your life might look like this:

- **8:30 a.m.: Your daughter refuses to eat more than a few bites of her oatmeal and berries.** You worry that she's missing an opportunity to get the whole grains and fruit she needs.

- **9:30 a.m.: Your daughter asks you to bake a batch of chocolate muffins (some people call these "cupcakes").** You think to yourself, "If I make chocolate muffins, she might eat them with milk, and milk has protein and calcium. I'll put some fruit on the plate, too." You get out the muffin mix.

- **10:15 a.m.: The muffins are done. You serve a muffin with a glass of milk and a side of pineapple slices, along with a chicken nugget for protein. Your daughter eats the muffin and the nugget and leaves the milk and pineapple.** You think, "Hooray! Protein!

- **11:30 a.m.: You step out of the shower to find two empty muffin liners sitting on the kitchen table.** You sigh.

- **Noon: Your daughter says she isn't hungry for lunch.** You know why!

- **2:00 p.m.: Your husband comes home from work early and offers to take your daughter out for ice cream.** You say, "I wish she'd eat something more nutritious than ice cream . . . but she hasn't had any calcium, and she can always use more protein. Ice cream has both. Make sure she eats every last lick!"

Nutritionistas have great intentions; they just want their kids to consume the necessary nutrients. This concern is reasonable. All kids need healthy food to grow, and some children, especially those who are underweight, need careful monitoring.

But Nutritionistas are *so* worried about nutrients that they become impatient, and that's what trips them up. They offer healthy foods, like oatmeal with berries, but if their kids pass them up, the Nutritionista panics. She thinks, "My kid needs more protein. More calcium. More nutrients." And she will do anything, even give her child chocolate muffins, chicken nuggets, and ice cream, if she thinks it will help even a little bit of nutrition make its way into her kid's stomach.

A Nutritionista thinks of her child as an unusually picky and difficult eater. "If you had my child, you'd understand why I have to make chocolate muffins for breakfast," the Nutritionista says. But most of the Nutritionistas I know have kids who are no different from anyone else's. It's just that the Nutritionista has taught her children that if they hold out against eating new or healthy food long enough, Mom will come to the rescue with some of their favorite dishes. Sometimes, though, Nutritionistas really do have kids who are very sensitive to variations in the way food tastes or to different textures. This makes life more challenging, but these kids need help learning how to overcome their sensitivities. Serving them a menu of cupcakes and ice cream only reinforces the problems they have learning to eat right.

How can Nutritionistas change their ways? I recommend finding a safeguard that helps them relax about nutrition. For many parents, this is a multivitamin. For others, the safeguard is sneaking some fruit into a milkshake that you serve once a day or finding another way to slip nutrition into your child's favorite food. I usually discourage parents from being sneaky, but sometimes this is the only thing that gives Nutritionistas the confidence to overcome their hang-ups and make changes.

I saw this work for my Nutritionista client Ellen. Her son refused everything but hot dogs (protein!) and pizza (calcium!), and he wouldn't eat those unless he could watch Elmo at the same time. Whenever she considered turning off the tube, Ellen panicked that Jeremy would simply stop eating and not get any nutrition at all. Then she decided to give Jeremy a vitamin pill in the mornings. In the evening, she held her breath, turned off the television, and served a slightly different meal. Jeremy howled, but the vitamin safeguard gave Ellen the strength to endure a few nights of protest. In a couple of days, he began to eat a more varied diet, Elmo not included.

THE FOOD POLICE

Do you see yourself in any of these statements?

- My kids aren't allowed to eat candy.

- My kids aren't allowed anything with high fructose corn syrup, additives, or artificial dyes.

- I let my children eat cakes, cookies, and muffins, but only the kind *I* bake, because I know they're made with whole grains, applesauce, and flax seeds.

If you're nodding your head, you may be a badge-carrying member of the Food Police.

The Food Police worry about nutrition as much as the Nutritionistas do, but they solve the problem in a different way. Whereas Nutritionistas are willing to overlook "bad" nutrients like sugar as long as their children are taking in "good" nutrients like calcium, the Food Police don't accept these justifications. They expect their children to get their nutrients from whole, unprocessed, healthy foods.

That's a great food philosophy, except that the Food Police take it too far. The Food Police *never* take a day off. They're on the beat 24/7, always patrolling the kitchen to make sure their kids eat right. In the homes of the Food Police, meals are well-intentioned exercises in obedience and control.

"Wait," you might be saying. "You don't know the whole story. My child gets completely hyper when she eats sugar. Food dyes make my child start acting out. Children are especially sensitive to pesticides."

Let me say: (1) I believe you. (2) I'm sure they do. (3) You're right.

There are lots of legitimate reasons to be concerned about the foods our kids eat, and there may be good reasons you're concerned about the foods eaten by *your* child in particular. For the most part, I'm with you. I'm just saying . . . be careful. If you find yourself using lots of pressure tactics or becoming very restrictive, your hard work could backfire. If you push them to eat predetermined amounts of food, your kids might stop trusting their bodies to tell them when they're hungry and when they're full. If you completely withhold other foods, like sweets, your kids will never learn the skill of eating treats in moderation. And if your kitchen table is a battlefield, they will associate food with stress.

My client Jennifer was headed for all of these problems. Jennifer wanted her family to eat organic, whole foods without a whiff of junkiness about them. She had been arguing with her sons, who wanted to snack on applesauce and fruit cups while Jennifer insisted on apples.

In Jennifer's defense, it is true that eating an actual apple is better for kids than eating applesauce. And fruit cups that are processed and sweetened can be pretty close to junk food. But as I talked to Jennifer, it became clear that there was a troublesome pattern developing here. The family wasn't just battling over apples versus applesauce; every meal was an arena for argument. "Eat your vegetables. No, you can't get down from the table; you've barely eaten. No, we're not having dessert tonight. Eat your vegetables!"

I proposed that Jennifer let her kids have a little more control. She started by stocking a snack drawer with granola and dried fruit—items Jennifer was comfortable with—as well as the applesauce and fruit cups that her kids craved. Finally, I recommended that Jennifer tell her sons that they could each select one item from the snack drawer every day. She was not to second-guess their decisions.

The boys were remarkably and instantly happy, not just because they suddenly got to snack on items they really wanted but because they were given more control over their eating. As it turns out, the boys didn't eat as much of the "bad stuff" as Jennifer had originally feared, and that helped Jennifer loosen up on the pressure and restriction she'd been using at mealtimes. It wasn't long before the boys were starting to eat the way Jennifer wanted (lots of vegetables, not too many desserts, a rotation through healthy and not-so-healthy snacks), and their control struggles cooled down.

NURTURERS

Nurturers feed to show love. We (yes, I'm a Nurturer) are motivated by how feeding others makes *us* feel. And boy, does it feel good. I get a rush from giving my daughter cookies. It makes me feel fantastic to give her cake. And while I'm confessing, nothing beats giving her ice cream.

When I provide a wholesome meal—complete with a salad and

vegetables—I feel like a good mother. But when I give my daughter the treats she adores, I feel even better. I feel like I'm directly transferring love from my heart to hers. It's like hooking up an IV of happiness. My daughter lights up when she gets these goodies, and making her happy makes me happy. Actually, it makes me ecstatic!

There's a drawback to my cookies = love equation, though. It makes it difficult for me to teach my daughter one of the most important things she needs to learn in order to eat right: how often to eat different kinds of foods. Treats should be offered (and eaten) occasionally. But I love my daughter more than occasionally. I love her every day! That causes a conflict for me. I really want my daughter to learn that food is food, that treats are treats, and that love is a feeling. Mixing up her food and my feelings leads to all kinds of eating struggles, ones I would like to spare her. Yet it's still hard for me not to overfeed my daughter her favorites.

I know I'm not alone in my nurturing tendencies. Think of all those grandmothers who live to give. Typically excellent cooks, these Nurturers have good intentions, but they may not get the best results. That was Beatrice's situation. Her Italian mother-in-law was constantly pushing pasta, meatballs, and an assortment of other yummy treats onto the plate of seventeen-month-old George. Some kids would respond by overeating and confusing food with a grandmother's love. In George's case, the opposite happened; he felt so much pressure to eat that he responded by eating less. A lot less. And each day that his grandmother responded to George's resistance by showing more love with more food, George felt more pressure. The solution was to start serving significantly smaller portions. When George's grandmother began pulling back on the portions, George's eating began to improve.

Some people become Nurturers because they believe in what I call the *kids and cookies culture*. This is a belief that childhood is a special time, when children should have a free pass to eat whatever cookies and candy they want. Implicit in this line of thinking are two ideas. One is that treats are the essence of a happy childhood, distilled and captured in candy form. The other is that kids have a protected period of time when how they eat doesn't matter. And to look at many kids it seems true: They're not overweight, and some even eat their vegetables! My friend Jonathan, who is a kids-and-cookies kind of Nurturer, once summed up his attitude toward the candy his kids consumed this way: "They might as well eat it now, while they can, because they're not going to be able to eat it when they're older."

Unfortunately, loading goodies onto the plate teaches children the wrong habits. You don't want your kids confusing love with casseroles or candy, because kids who do will have trouble changing those habits later in life.

COMFORTERS

When your child skins her knee, do you whip out a cookie? If you do, you're probably a Comforter. Unlike Nurturers, who use food to express their love, Comforters use food to wipe away tears and to banish any difficult emotions their children are feeling.

It's easy to confuse Comforters with Nurturers because they both use food to cope with feelings.

- You're a Nurturer if you use food to *show your* feelings.

- You're a Comforter if you use food to *stop their* feelings.

Now, while I am a Nurturer, I am definitely not a Comforter. That's why I so vividly remember the first time someone tried to soothe my crying child with a sweet. We were at the doctor's office. My daughter was crying from a vaccination, and the nurse offered her a lollipop.

Having watched both my mother's constant struggle with food and her premature death from obesity-related issues, I am hyperattuned to the problems associated with using food to soothe the soul. And so, on that day at the doctor's office, I whisked the lollipop away from the nurse before my daughter could see it. I soothed her with hugs and kisses, and then, only after my daughter had recovered from the trauma, did I offer up the lollipop.

You see, I wasn't against the lollipop. I was against teaching my daughter to eat for emotional reasons. You might think young children are immune to eating for emotional reasons, but they're not. It's actually surprisingly easy to teach children to comfort themselves with food. Those toddlers who are old enough to sleep through the night but who wake up multiple times for milk? Chances are they're not really hungry. Instead, they've already learned to rely on milk for comfort.

If you frequently fix boo-boos with brownies or repair hurt feelings with cookies, then watch out: You might be teaching your children to soothe their souls with sweets. This is a problem because children who use food to deal with emotions end up overeating. This might not be a big deal if kids responded to stress by eating a bunch of broccoli, but they don't. In a crisis, kids turn to chocolate, cake, and ice cream, just like adults do.

It gets worse. The problem with teaching children to eat for emotional reasons isn't just that they use distress as a cue to eat. It's that they also end up confusing the *feeling* of distress with the *feeling* of hunger. This makes children more likely to respond to negative feelings with food, not because the food makes them feel better emotionally but because the food makes them feel full.

The Comforter solution is straightforward. Rather than automatically handing out sweets when your kids melt down, ask yourself what they *really* need. A hug? A nap? A snack? Follow up with the appropriate response. True, there are going to be times when you get it wrong. It's also true that some emotional eating is unavoidable. But consciously parenting kids around food means minimizing the times we use food as a tool.

ONWARD!

If you didn't see yourself in any of the profiles I just described, guess what? You're not off the hook. Every single one of us struggles with *something*. If you're a parent, I guarantee you've got an issue. I've covered only the most common ones. But maybe you're a rare bird. Maybe you're more like a:

- **Time Buyer:** The kind of parent who *always* has cookies on hand to distract your kids so you can read, work, talk on the phone, shop, cook, and think with a little peace and quiet.

- **Principled Junk Eater:** A parent who loves fast food and sweets; these parents would like to teach their children better habits but don't want to be hypocrites. ("How can I ask her to eat vegetables when I can't stand them?")

- **Rewarder:** The sort of parent who thinks kids deserve treats for every success, no matter how small; rewarders pass out cake and cookies for good report cards, good soccer games, and good days at school.

There are probably as many hang-ups as there are parents. The point of identifying your issue isn't to make you feel bad. I'm a Nurturer at heart. I know plenty of successful parents who are recovering Nutritionistas, Comforters, and members of the Food Police.

What do we have in common? We've all figured out our weak spots and the ways we're most likely to sabotage our own efforts. Now we're stronger and more effective. Time and time again, I've found that when parents recognize their feeding hang-ups, they can produce deep and lasting transformations to the way their children eat because they stop teaching their children so many unintended lessons. No matter what your hang-up, know this: Nothing is too big or too bad for you to conquer.

We all have hopes and dreams for our children. For most of us, they involve wanting our kids to be happy and healthy eaters. In Part Two, I outline some practical steps you can take right now to make that happen.

Part Two

. . .

Teaching Habits

The Big Fix

The goal of the teaching approach is simple: to teach children the three habits of proportion, variety, and moderation—in other words, how to eat a variety of foods in moderation and in proportion to their health benefits.

But here's what happens at your house: You want your child to eat dinner. He doesn't. At least not that load of disgusting, yucky, awful-looking slop you so thoughtlessly put on his plate. Instead of eating, he's sitting with arms crossed and giving you a defiant stare. How are you supposed to teach proportion, variety, or moderation under these conditions?

You can't. Not yet. Before you can change *what* your kids eat, you have to change *how* you and your kids interact around food. In this chapter, I suggest a new pattern of interactions. These interactions will help you leave the nutrition mindset behind. They'll free you up to teach about habits and free your kids to learn them. They create a structure that cuts the food dramas and sets your child up to succeed at learning proportion, variety, and moderation.

I call this structure The Big Fix. The Big Fix won't make all your family's food problems go away, but I bet it will cut them in half. (If you are reading this book before your children are old enough to have food problems, The Big Fix will prevent a lot of them from happening in the first place.) The Big Fix doesn't have to do with getting your kids to eat things they don't want. It doesn't ask you to serve anything new. It doesn't even ask you to start teaching the habits of proportion, variety, and moderation. But once you have The Big Fix in place, teaching those habits will be a whole lot easier.

STUCK IN A STRUCTURE

When you have a nutrition mindset, it's *so easy* to get stuck in behaviors that don't work. That's what the first part of this book was all about. Parents who are focused on nutrition will almost always fall into traps and give too much voice to hang-ups that reinforce their kids' limited food preferences and poor eating patterns. If this has happened to you, it's not your fault. It's just the inevitable outcome of the nutrition mindset.

Those traps and hang-ups can develop into a frustrating routine. In sociology, a repeating pattern of relationships is called a *structure*. Structures shape how people act; when a structure is in place among a group of people, you can predict many of their interactions. If you are having trouble getting your kids to eat right, stop for a minute to think about whether you are locked into a structure that isn't working. I've seen plenty of parents who try hard to improve how their kids eat, but most of the time they draw from the same stock of strategies. "Just taste it." "Two more bites." "If you want some dessert . . ." The kids have a pattern, too. They respond with essentially the same set of reactions. They dawdle. Take two teeny bites. Scream no. In the end, things may change a little, but because the parents and kids have conformed to their assigned scripts, they wind up basically in the same place where they started. If you really want to change how your kids eat, you have to change the structure.

Parents are always surprised when I can describe the dance they are doing with their children before they tell me all of the details of their particular tango. I'm not clairvoyant; I have just had a lot of practice looking for patterns in how people interact. Because I don't get caught up in the nuances of any immediate meal, I am able to examine the family's eating structure to determine which elements are working and which elements aren't. That's what happened when Steven came to see me about the problems he was having with his nine-year-old daughter, Morgan. One issue they'd been fighting over was whether Morgan had to eat breakfast. Steven was worn down. He had run out of ideas.

"Let me guess what's going on," I said to Steven. "Every morning you walk into the kitchen with a knot in your stomach, wondering how you are going to get Morgan to eat breakfast today. Morgan walks in with her defenses up, ready to do battle. Am I right?"

Steven nodded.

I continued: "You offer Morgan eggs. She says no. You offer her toast. She says she's not hungry. You say she has to eat something before going to school. Morgan says she'll be fine. You keep offering her anything you can think of until, eventually, you run out of steam. Then, either you let Morgan go to school without eating breakfast or you end up offering Morgan something she can't resist, something like a doughnut. She's won. And you? You feel frustrated, annoyed, and defeated."

Steven agreed. The scenario I described was spot on. But here's what happened next. With a little more probing, we discovered that

Morgan really *was* hungry in the morning. In fact, she was so hungry that on the days Steven didn't give in by handing Morgan a sweet treat, Morgan ate her bagged lunch as she walked to school. That's how Morgan could afford to challenge Steven on breakfast every day; she had a quick and easy backup. But, as I'm sure you can imagine, eating her lunch at eight o'clock in the morning was causing a problem for Morgan when lunchtime rolled around. Things had to change.

Steven wondered if, perhaps, the problem was that Morgan didn't really like to eat breakfast foods. It's true that there are advantages to breaking out of the breakfast-food rut, but Steven had already bent over backward to offer Morgan many different kinds of breakfast options; my guess was that in this case, the problem was only partly about the food. I was more interested in the fact that Morgan had become accustomed to pushing back against Steven's insistence that she eat. It was almost certainly the case that when Morgan walked into the kitchen she never even stopped to evaluate how hungry she was. Instead, because Steven was being controlling, Morgan slipped into an automatic response: She was controlling right back.

On the surface, it may not seem like Steven was being controlling. Compared to parents who make their children eat their vegetables, finish all the food on their plates, or never allow their kids to eat sweets and treats, Steven's morning routine seems downright solicitous: "Do you want to eat toast?" "Do you want to eat eggs?" But Steven was being controlling because he never accepted Morgan's assertion that she didn't want to eat *anything*. Every morning, Steven steamrolled right over her protests.

Of course, Steven had good reason to be concerned about whether Morgan ate breakfast. We all know how important breakfast is. But pushing Morgan to eat every morning wasn't, in fact, teaching her the importance of starting the day off with a nourishing meal. It was teaching her something else. That "something else" was the problem.

Steven thought he was teaching one lesson when he was really teaching a different one. Did Morgan know that her father wanted her to have a healthy start to her day? Sure. But that was not her primary takeaway. The main message Morgan was learning was that the only way to have any control over what she ate was to fight for it. In her house, control over food was something to be contested. In fact, control was like a ball that she and her father threw back and forth. First he had the ball, then she did.

The gap between the lesson parents think they are teaching and the lessons their children are actually learning is where most problems flourish. Every morning when Steven used his "breakfast is important" speech he hoped that, *today*, Morgan would finally *get it*. When she didn't seem to get it (because nothing changed), Steven responded by repeating his message, sometimes making the speech a little bit longer, sometimes saying it a little bit louder. What Steven couldn't see, though, was that Morgan *was* getting the message. The message she was getting, though, was different from the one Steven intended. Morgan was learning that eating is all about control. Moreover, because each fight unwittingly reinforced the message mix-up, every morning Steven and Morgan became increasingly entrenched in their respective positions. It was a classic example of a system that teaches the wrong lessons.

ONE EXTREME TO THE OTHER

When systems don't work, it's usually because the parents are either overly controlling or overly permissive. Which parenting style you gravitate toward is shaped by your basic personality. It is also shaped, in large part, by whatever issue is holding you hostage. Hunger Avoiders, Nutritionistas, and It's-Just-a-Phasers, for example, lean toward being permissive parents; the Food Police are more controlling.

But we all have the potential to parent from either extreme—or from both of them. That is what was happening to Steven. Steven was alternating between pressuring Morgan (by insisting that she eat breakfast) and giving up (by capitulating and letting Morgan eat whatever she wanted). Neither extreme worked. Here's why.

Pushy or controlling parents (sometimes called *authoritarian parents*) exert too much control over what and how much their children eat. Kids who are naturally compliant will yield to the pressure, but in the process they also learn to eat more food than they desire (because their parents tell them to clean their plates), to dislike food they are being pressured to eat, and to prefer foods they are being denied. These are not the lessons their parents intend. When children are naturally more oppositional or defiant, an authoritarian parenting style has a different effect. It teaches these kids to lock horns. They think, "If you push me, I'm going to push back." In the process, it also teaches defiant children another counterproductive lesson: to dislike the food they are fighting about.

Permissive parents tend to allow kids to eat whatever they want, but strangely enough, they also teach their children to fight about food. Permissive parents offer to make special meals for their children, let them regularly substitute foods during meals, and give them easy access to unhealthy snacks. As a result, permissive parents typically have kids whose diets are filled with lots of treats and favorites and relatively few fruits and vegetables. But most permissive parents don't give up on healthy eating entirely. They keep trying to get their children to eat more produce, they do their best to

introduce new foods, and, as with Steven, they reinforce the importance of eating meals. What happens, though, when their children
start to complain? Permissive parents persist for a while, but they
eventually concede, like Steven did. What do kids learn from this
kind of interaction? That if they complain and whine and act difficult, it is only a matter of time before they get what they want. That
knowledge keeps the conflict going.

Many of the parents I know go back and forth between an authoritarian and a permissive style of parenting around food because
they (mistakenly) believe that these are the only two choices they
have. When one style fails to produce the right effects, parents flip
to the other style. However, when they find out that that approach
doesn't work any better—their kids *still* aren't trying new foods,
and *still* aren't eating more vegetables—parents ultimately end up
reverting to their original position. Back and forth they go. Sound
familiar?

The solution is to find the middle ground. Researchers call this
parenting style *authoritative*. Authoritative parents are successful
because they are able to create an eating structure that is firm but
flexible. They do this by setting limits while simultaneously staying
warm and responsive to their children's needs. Kids need boundaries to learn to eat right, but they also need the freedom to explore
and contribute to their own eating decisions. A certain amount of
parental direction and control is necessary, but that control can't be
overwhelming.

Toeing the line between a pushy and a permissive parenting
style sounds more difficult than it is. You just have to think beyond
the immediate meal to consider your children's broad eating
patterns; to look at the forest rather than the trees. I told Steven
that the most effective way I know to create a supportive structure
for eating is for parents to set a few simple guidelines around when

The Pressure Perception

Parents often don't think they are pressuring their children, but pressure, like beauty, is in the eye of the beholder. When a team of Pennsylvania State University researchers asked a group of parents and their five-year-old daughters about pressure, only 26 percent of the parents said they pressured their daughter to eat. In contrast, 61 percent of the girls said their parents used pressure tactics to get them to eat. That's an astonishing divide.

and how foods are chosen, and then to let their kids participate in many of the choices. That's what I call The Big Fix.

THE BIG FIX

The Big Fix is surprisingly simple. It lets you take down your old structure, the one that isn't working for your family. Then it builds up a new structure based on three rules:

- You decide *when* your children eat. You do this by identifying Eating Zones.

- You decide *what* your children eat. By implementing the Rotation Rule, you'll form the foundation for good eating habits without having to introduce new or disliked foods.

- Within the framework of the first two rules, you systematically allow your children some control. You give them choices.

Doesn't sound revolutionary enough to change how things are going in your house? It is. The Big Fix works because it creates a firm but flexible structure that enables you to set limits while still remaining warm and responsive to your children's needs. Yes! The Big Fix is authoritative parenting in action.

The first two rules give you a clear and consistent way to be firm about when and what your children eat. Then sharing control enables you to be warm and responsive to your children's needs and desires. What about the three habits of proportion, variety, and moderation? With The Big Fix, you don't directly teach those habits, not yet. But you'll find that The Big Fix points your family in the right direction.

TEAR DOWN YOUR OLD STRUCTURE

Before you can build your new structure, you have to take down your old one. Why bother with this step? Why not just switch from one approach to the other? Because if you are locked in conflict with your child, *nothing* you do is going to work. If you and your child are in opposition when it comes to food, your child will be primed to resist all your efforts, no matter what they are.

Remember Steven? The only way he would ever get Morgan to eat breakfast without a fight would be if the two of them stopped seeing each other as adversaries. They had to start seeing themselves as partners who were working toward a mutual goal. For that to happen, Steven and Morgan would need a cooling-off period. Once the tension was gone, they could start fresh, reinventing the way they interacted. Right now, though, Steven and Morgan needed to push the reset button.

You probably know exactly what you need to do to reduce the tension in your household. Most parents do. It's this:

Stop asking your children to change how they eat!

I'm not kidding. This is precisely what you need to do. For just a little while, I want you to tap into your inner permissive parent. Do you and your child bicker over whether he should eat at the table? Let him dine on the sofa. If you usually sigh and complain about having to make your child the same grilled cheese sandwich every day for lunch, make the sandwich with a smile on your face. Whatever it is you're arguing over, just stop. Stop measuring out the number of bites your child has to eat before getting dessert. Stop begging your child to try the fish. Stop, stop, stop. Stop for about a week or two, until you sense that the food tension has eased.

In Steven's case, I asked him, "What would get Morgan to stop fighting with you about food?" He knew the answer right away: giving her something sugary for breakfast. I suggested that he take Morgan to the grocery store so she could pick out any food she wanted.

"Any food she wants?" Steven asked. He looked unhappy. "She'll go straight for the sweetened cereals."

I explained that this step was a temporary measure—a peace offering—designed to reduce tension. Steven was skeptical, but he decided to give it a shot. As Steven expected, Morgan ended up choosing a sweetened cereal at the grocery store, though one that was not as bad as Steven originally feared. Having "her" cereal got Morgan excited about eating breakfast. Each morning, instead of dragging her feet, Morgan came bounding into the kitchen, eager to dig in and eat.

As you might have guessed, Morgan's newfound enthusiasm for eating breakfast had a big effect on Steven. She willingly ate breakfast, and he began to relax, confident in the knowledge that he was no longer sending his daughter off to school on an empty stomach. (Of course, Steven still held out hope for the healthier breakfast, and I assured him that was coming.) Within a week or so the tension between Steven and Morgan was completely gone. They were ready to start The Big Fix.

GET YOUR KIDS ON BOARD

I'll get into the details of The Big Fix in just a minute, but first I want to give you a key to success. If there is one thing you can do to make sure The Big Fix works, it's this: Don't keep it a secret. Talk to your kids before you implement any of the three rules. Talk to your kids *while* you implement the new rules. And keep on talking to them until the new structure comes naturally to everyone.

If you don't talk to your kids about the changes you are making, your system will seem arbitrary to them. Not only does an arbitrary environment feel unfair to kids, but it also suggests that every decision is up for grabs. "Why can't I have another snack right now?" "How many bites of eggs do I have to eat before I can get a waffle?" "Can I have a waffle if I promise I'll eat eggs tomorrow?" This way of interacting trains your kids to become excellent lawyers one day, but it inflames the food fight right now.

When you make your rules clear and consistent, a lot of conflict ends. So once you're ready to begin The Big Fix, take the time to explain the new rules—no matter how old (or how young) your kids are. Make both your long- and short-term goals transparent; it will help your children learn the right lessons. Let your kids know what you'll expect from them, and ask for their feedback and questions. Remember, you and your kids are on the same team. But your kids can't cooperate with your new structure if they don't know what it is.

THE BIG FIX RULE 1:
DECIDE *WHEN* YOUR CHILD EATS

One reason Morgan had been able to engage in the breakfast struggle was that no matter how hungry she was in the morning, she always knew that she could eat her lunch on the way to school. In other words, Morgan had no incentive to eat breakfast because there was another "breakfast" (her lunch) waiting in the wings.

A lot of families suffer from this kind of cycle: Kids don't eat particularly well at meals, so they gorge on snacks. Then, because they are full from snacks, these kids don't eat particularly well at meals. It is a cycle that parents recognize but find hard to break. I am not surprised, because when parents try to solve the problem, they often use a controlling approach, cutting snacks out altogether. But when parents try to starve out their kids, the effort almost always fails. The kids either get so hungry they have meltdowns or dig in their heels and hold out for what feels like—to the parents, at least—forever. Even when parents do triumph in this battle of wills, it's a false win, because the family control struggle becomes even more entrenched.

Let's see who breaks first is not a great paradigm for parenting.

Instead of trying to starve out your kids, try a more authoritative (not authoritarian) approach. Provide a reasonable time structure for both snacks and meals. This is what Eating Zones are for. These zones are regular blocks of time that you create—one for each daily meal and snack. On any given day, you can choose one specific time during each Eating Zone when you will offer something to eat.

Eating Zones help you avoid constant on-demand grazing, but they do not snap you into a rigid schedule. To create your Eating

Zones, look at your typical day to see when you normally provide meals and snacks. Account for variables, such as naps, outings, school, or your work schedule. Evaluate when your child is usually hungry, when she is too tired or too hungry to eat, and any other circumstances that affect her appetite.

Using this information, create several blocks of time each day that you will set aside for meals and snacks. This should feel like a schedule, but a pretty loose one. Below is a sample day of how Eating Zones worked for one of my clients with a toddler. Your family's Eating Zones will probably look a little different.

This family would serve breakfast any time between 7:30 and 9:00, morning snack any time between 10:00 and 11:00, lunch between noon and 1:00 . . . you get the idea. Pick a time to serve food during whatever Eating Zone you're in, and then you're done until the next Eating Zone comes around. With this structure, you can be flexible about when you serve food, but there are also clear times when food is *not* going to be available. You can think of these times as *No*-Eating Zones.

That's it. You create opportunities for eating, but let your children choose whether and how much to eat.

SAMPLE EATING ZONES

Choose any time between . . .	To serve
7:30 and 9:00	Breakfast
10:00 and 11:00	Morning snack
12:00 and 1:00	Lunch
3:00 and 4:30	Afternoon snack
5:30 and 7:00	Dinner

The Eating Zones are designed to let you respond to your child's individual hunger signals. Let's say you're on an Eating Zone schedule like the one just given. Your daughter refuses breakfast when you serve it at 8:00 a.m. but then says she is hungry at 8:30. Under this plan, you *don't* tell her, "Tough! You missed breakfast, and now you have to wait for lunch!" (That's controlling.) And you *don't* rush to provide her with a snack or substitute breakfast right away. (That would be permissive.) Instead, you can be authoritative. You can commiserate and then offer a snack at the very beginning of the next Eating Zone—at 10:00. That way, she experiences the hunger that is a natural consequence of skipping breakfast, but she's not hungry for all that long, and she's never truly starving. And if your child eats a *huge* breakfast, you can wait until the end of the next Eating Zone to serve morning snack.

Here's how one family explained Eating Zones to their child:

Sweetie, meals have not been so much fun lately. We've been trying to make you eat your food at mealtimes, and you've been unhappy about that. Right? Well, we have decided that starting tonight we are not going to make you eat at meals anymore. In fact, we are never going to make you eat anything ever again. You are a big girl now, and we think you can figure this out for yourself. Instead, we are going to put together a plan for meals and snacks. Every day we are going to give you breakfast, lunch, and dinner as usual. But we are also going to give you a morning snack and an afternoon snack, too. How does that sound?

But here's the thing—if you decide that you don't want to eat anything or that you want to stop eating before your tummy has had enough food, you might get hungry. And that's OK, too, because there will always be another snack or meal in a little while.

You will have to wait for that snack or mealtime to come around, though. I know you can do this. If you are hungry, come tell us, and we'll tell you how much time you have to wait. It might be hard at first, but I know you can do it.

Feeling nervous about this conversation? Asking a hungry child to wait before eating may seem as if it's inviting *more* conflict, not less. (And more conflict might be terrifying if you're a Peacemaker.) And you might get some pushback, but only in the beginning. Once your children learn that they have a dependable eating routine, they will embrace it without much fuss.

For some parents, especially Hunger Avoiders, it's very difficult to stop telling their children to eat more at meals. But they have to, even if their children make mistakes by undereating. Knowing that there will be times when they won't be able to eat creates an incentive for children to eat when food is available. Moreover, before children can voluntarily choose *to* eat, they need the freedom to choose *not* to eat.

Consider Unconventional Eating Times

When you evaluate your child's daily schedule, it is often instrumental to break out of the idea that meals need to occur during conventional time periods. To illustrate what I mean, let me tell you about Tucker.

Tucker is a bright and engaging three-year-old boy. His mother, Nell, was frustrated by an afternoon pattern of hunger-induced meltdowns, followed by a period of nonstop grazing, and then a struggle over dinner.

Nell told me that the problem was caused by Tucker's preschool schedule. The program ran daily from noon until 2:30, right when

TUCKER'S TYPICAL SCHEDULE

8:00	Morning milk
9:30	Breakfast
11:00	Lunch (always refused)
11:30	Leave for school
Noon–2:30	School
2:30	Snack offered while traveling home (always refused)
4:00–7:00	Grazing
7:00	Dinner (always refused)

most kids are eating lunch. Nell had tried offering Tucker lunch at around 11:00, but he always refused to eat. But then, she reported, he would be so hungry when she picked him up after preschool that he would fall apart. Nell would offer Tucker a snack, but it was impossible for him to eat until he calmed down, which didn't happen until around 4:00. At that point, Tucker would start grazing, all the way up until dinnertime. Of course, that meant Tucker typically refused to eat dinner.

Nell wanted to know how she could stave off the afternoon tantrums. We looked at Tucker's schedule and had a few insights. By drinking a large glass of milk first thing in the morning—something many young children do because they are hungry and thirsty and find milk comforting—Tucker was putting into place a domino effect of off-kilter eating. The milk filled Tucker sufficiently that he didn't want breakfast until mid-morning; the late breakfast meant he didn't want an early lunch; Tucker would get hungry during school, and by the time he was picked up, he was starving; tantrums and then an afternoon of grazing subsequently ruined dinner.

I recommended that Nell make the following changes to Tucker's schedule:

- A small morning milk and light breakfast first thing in the morning

- Early lunch

- Small snack while in transit before and after school

- Early dinner if Tucker is hungry early, later dinner if he is not

When you look at these Eating Zones, I know it seems like a lot of eating. But like many children, Tucker had three meals and two snacks—it's just that his lunch and first snack were at somewhat unusual times. There were also plenty of periods during the day when he was *not* eating. Because he wasn't grazing between 4:00 and dinner, he actually had fewer snacks on this plan than he had before. Almost as soon as Nell began the Eating Zones, Tucker began eating more at lunch and dinner, and his tantrums ended.

TUCKER'S NEW EATING ZONES

7:00–8:30	Small morning milk and light breakfast
10:30–11:30	Lunch
11:30–noon	Snack while traveling to school
Noon–2:30	School
2:30–3:30	Snack
4:30–7:00	Dinner

Tucker's schedule is not right for everyone. You need to figure out what will work in your home. Do you have to fix an early breakfast so that everyone can get to daycare and work? Does your child do better with a snack before bed? Two snacks in the morning? Do your kids burn through so many calories with late-afternoon sports that it's better to serve a full meal after school and a hearty snack in the evening? Consider your child's needs—and your reality—and align your Eating Zones to suit them both.

Serving a very early dinner is another unconventional move that worked for Tucker and is great for many kids. Young children are often hungry for dinner around 4:30. Dinner is not typically served, though, until later, and so children start snacking. When dinner finally arrives, the kids are full. And because snacks are rarely dinner-quality food, the kids are full of *junk*. Then parents spend dinner trying to force healthy food into a child with no appetite:

> PARENT: *Eat some more broccoli.*
> CHILD: *I'm not hungry.*
> PARENT: *That's because you ate so many crackers! You need something healthy. Eat some more broccoli.*
> CHILD: *I'm not hungry!*

When you move dinner earlier to match when children are hungry, you avoid excessive snacking and dramatically reduce the dinnertime struggle. If the adults want to have their own dinner later, that's fine. Your child can join you for conversation and dessert.

Remember to Reduce Tension First!

Let's return to Steven and Morgan. Steven spent a few weeks reducing tension around food by putting an end to his wheedling, suggesting, offering, sighing, and lecturing during breakfast. Instead he clamped his mouth shut and allowed Morgan to eat the sugary cereal she wanted. This step was difficult for Steven, but it paid off. It made Eating Zones easy. Because she was eating breakfast, Morgan no longer snacked on her packed lunch during the walk to school. From there, Morgan's school naturally imposed Eating Zones with clearly delineated eating and noneating times. Her father served a snack after school, dinner in the early evening, and a light snack before bed. Soon Morgan's eating settled into a meal-centered routine.

I know, Morgan was eating a junky breakfast. Her other food choices weren't so great, either. Steven and I would work on that next. But sometimes, you have to take a step backward before you can move ahead.

Before you do anything else, you have to reduce tension. Until you do, everything else you do will feel like a showdown.

THE BIG FIX RULE 2: THE ROTATION RULE

Now that you've structured when your kids eat, it's time for the next phase of The Big Fix: You'll build a structure for *what* your children eat. You do this with the Rotation Rule.

The Rotation Rule couldn't be simpler:

Never serve the same food (except milk) two days in a row.

This is a very basic principle, but it will change your life. That's no exaggeration. I've had parents tell me that after they began using the Rotation Rule, their kids started being less fussy; they asked to taste new foods; and some even started to eat vegetables!

The secret to the Rotation Rule is that it lets parents create a straightforward guideline for how food choices are made that is clear and easy to explain to even the youngest children. But it's a guideline, not a whip. Even though parents are in charge of what foods can be served, there's enough flexibility in the system to offer children lots of choices. Remember, *the combination of structure and flexibility is the magic formula used by authoritative parents*. It dissolves the control struggles that are the hidden cause of most poor eating.

Plus, the Rotation Rule builds a foundation for changing what your kids eat. If you serve the same foods every day, your kids will come to expect the same foods every day. But the Rotation Rule creates a different expectation. With the Rotation Rule, you don't serve any new or disliked foods. Let me say that again: *You don't serve any foods that your kids don't already eat willingly!* You just make sure that they don't eat the same food two days in a row. Your kids will stop expecting to have the exact same flavors and textures every day. In a small but profound way, they'll begin to *expect* more variety. And then they'll *accept* more variety. This acceptance comes quickly for some kids; for others, it takes more time. But it does happen. When variety becomes the new normal, your kids will naturally feel more comfortable eating different kinds of foods and tasting new ones. Eventually, variety becomes such an ingrained habit that your kids will think that having the same foods all the time is a little weird.

Make a List

Before you begin using the Rotation Rule, do a little prep work. Put together a list of all the foods your children willingly eat. Include everything they eat for meals and snacks—and I mean everything, even it feels embarrassing. Leave off all the foods you *wish* your children would eat but won't unless you resort to threats. The resulting list is a valuable document. It tells you all the foods you can use when you're implementing the Rotation Rule. No matter how limited your kids' diet or how oddball their preferences, the Rotation Rule can meet you where you are.

Consider compiling this list with your children. Although you're the project leader, they are your team members. Invite your kids to work with you. You might be surprised by what they come up with, including foods you didn't think they liked as well as foods you might have forgotten. Some families have turned this into an arts and crafts project by having children cut out magazine images or draw pictures of foods they enjoy eating. Some post the list or the drawings in the kitchen to remind themselves of the foods available for rotation.

Tell Your Kids the Plan

Next, tell your kids about the Rotation Rule. Remember, it's crucial to tell your kids what's going on. You can say, "I'd like you to learn how to eat in a healthier way. I know this is hard. That is why we are going to start off easy. We're going to rotate through your favorite foods."

Then clarify those parts of the plan that are firm and those parts that are flexible. Try something like this:

We are going to have a rule, which is that we don't eat the same food two days in a row. You will have some choices, but you can't break the rule. For instance, tomorrow I will ask you if you want to eat cereal or waffles. But if you want a muffin, which you ate this morning, I'm going to tell you no. You will have to wait until the next day. Unless it is a very special occasion, we are going to stick to the rule of not eating the same food two days in a row.

Finally, give your children a chance to share their reactions and concerns. Listen closely to what your kids have to say. This is how you bring your children into their part of the process and give them a vested interest in a positive outcome. It is also your ticket to success. When you know what part of the plan might trip your child up, you can devise ways to correct and modify potential pitfalls *before* they occur.

Rotate!

Now it's time to launch the Rotation Rule into action. All you have to do is switch up what you serve from day to day so that no food (except milk) appears on the menu two days in a row. If your child had chicken nuggets for lunch yesterday, you can offer anything on the list today *but* chicken nuggets. If you serve cheese puffs for snack one day, they are off the menu for the next day. You are consciously rotating through the foods your children already accept, whatever those foods happen to be—even if they are unhealthy. Keep following the Rotation Rule until it becomes a solid, unquestionable part of your child's eating routine. At that point, you're ready to move on to teaching proportion (the topic of the next chapter).

Steven and Morgan had great success with the Rotation Rule. Steven decided to use the Rotation Rule only at breakfast, which was fine. He told Morgan that she could continue to have her sweetened cereal, as long as she didn't eat it two days in a row. On the other mornings she would have to find something else to eat. Morgan agreed, partly because she was no longer locked in a fight and partly because she was being given a measure of control.

When I checked back a few weeks later, Steven told me things were going really well. Morgan eagerly ate breakfast, and even though Steven wished Morgan would eat more food in the morning, he had kept silent. Furthermore, the Rotation Rule was working. Morgan ate "her" cereal as often as the rule permitted, but on the other days she elected to eat something such as yogurt and fruit. One morning she ate vegetable soup and bread. Steven was thrilled.

Some parents worry that the Rotation Rule will feel constraining. If that happens, get creative. Switch up how and when you serve the items on your list, and you'll find a new world of options. You don't have to stick to breakfast foods for breakfast, lunch foods for lunch, and dinner foods for dinner. You certainly don't have to stick to snack foods for snacks, because any food can fit that category. Serve pancakes for dinner. Have carrot sticks and dip, or even chicken nuggets, pasta, or bean and cheese burritos, at breakfast. Chicken and broccoli for snack. Or ask your kids to help you invent new food combinations. Does your child like cottage cheese, bananas, and jelly? Put them together and make a breakfast banana split. Anything goes!

But you don't have to go crazy. You could, for instance, serve cereal one morning, eggs the next morning, and pancakes the following morning. You could use a rotation that goes from oatmeal with bananas to toast with butter and then back to the oatmeal. If that would be too much change for your child, you could alternate between kinds of cereal (Cheerios, then Special K, then Frosted Mini-Wheats) or you could even create a rotation by altering toppings on the same cereal: oatmeal with bananas, followed by oatmeal with bananas and cinnamon, followed by oatmeal with bananas and brown sugar. It doesn't really matter what the rotation is as long as you incorporate as much difference as your child can easily tolerate (without making it so easy that he doesn't experience a rotation).

What if you've got a *really* picky eater, one who eats only eight different foods? Or six? Or four? In these cases, you probably can't avoid serving some of the same foods two days in a row. However, you can still use the Rotation Rule to introduce your child to the idea of variety. One toddler I worked with was extraordinarily cautious. She ate only a few foods and just two kinds of produce: peach puree mixed with oatmeal, and green beans. Her mother had no choice but to serve these foods every day because she wanted her daughter to eat at least some kind of fruit and some kind of vegetable each and every day. To keep the idea of variety going from meal to meal, her mother switched up when and how she served the items. For example, some days she served the peach puree and oatmeal mixture for lunch or dinner instead of for breakfast. Sometimes she offered the peach puree mixed into something else her daughter liked, such as rice. She also served the puree on its own, in a little bowl. In tough cases like these, it's perfectly OK to establish a rotation based on small differences. Your child will embrace variety more slowly than other kids might, but be patient. It will happen.

THE BIG FIX RULE 3: GIVE YOUR KIDS CHOICES

Giving your children some choices is the warm and responsive part of authoritative parenting. It honors your children's desire for control—and then redirects it into an arena where their choices will not undermine their habits. For instance, as long as you monitor the Rotation Rule, it does not matter whether your children eat apples or bananas today. If you have both fruits on hand, why not ask for your children's input?

Make it clear to your children that you are offering them choices within the structure you have established. Some of the specifics might be up for grabs—Would you like to eat your snack now or in fifteen minutes?—but the Rotation and Eating Zones are not.

Here are some ways to give your children choices that will continue to build good habits:

- When you're getting food ready, let your children choose between two options. Grilled cheese or turkey? Green peppers or carrots? (Be wary of the open-ended question "What do you want?" This usually leads to a pattern of the parent rejecting the child's choices until the child chooses something acceptable or the child endlessly choosing and then rechoosing.)

- Serve three or four different dishes—say, one meat and two vegetables—and ask your children to choose something from at least two of the dishes. Let them serve themselves from the serving bowls.

- Keep a selection of raw vegetables—string beans, cherry tomatoes, red peppers, anything your children eat—in bowls in the refrigerator to supplement meals. Bring them out at dinnertime and ask your children to eat anything from the meal you've prepared and/or anything they want from the bowls.

- Ask your children what they would like you to prepare for dinner. Give them two or three choices of main dishes *or* two or three choices of side dishes. When you do prepare their choices, make sure to remind them that you complied with their request.

- Allow your children to choose which plate, which seat, which utensils, or which glass they want.

- Ask whether they want their food cut in slices, cubes, or circles (but only when it's convenient for you to do so).

- At the grocery store, have your children pick out the packet of peas they want, the shape of pasta, the color of potato.

- When the family schedule allows, let your children choose when they eat their snacks and meals, as long as they stay within the Eating Zones.

Expanding your children's choices won't guarantee that they'll eat what you serve, but the more you redirect your children's desire for control into appropriate arenas, the less they'll fight with you about eating. Don't overdo it, though. Too many choices can be as unsettling for kids as none at all! One or two choices per meal are enough.

BE PREPARED FOR IT ALL TO FALL APART!

PARENT: *Your choices today are waffles or eggs. Which would you like?*

CHILD: *Toast!*

Expect that your children will challenge The Big Fix. If they don't challenge the Eating Zones, they'll challenge the Rotation Rule or the choices you give. Some will challenge *everything*. There may be pushback, meltdowns, and tantrums as your kids try to reestablish the old patterns. They are trying to figure out if this new structure is really as firm as you say it is.

Parents who respond to these challenges by calmly reinforcing the new rules will soon be rewarded. In a few days, kids will accept the new way of doing things. But when parents waver or capitulate, they send the message that they aren't very serious about the new rules. As soon as kids realize this, the new system fails. So be prepared for a little rebellion. Have a plan in mind so that you're not caught off guard.

When children challenge the structure, what I like to do is remind them of the rules while actively teaching them the ideas behind The Big Fix:

> PARENT: *Would you like waffles or eggs?*
>
> CHILD: *Toast!*
>
> PARENT: *You had toast yesterday. You can have toast again tomorrow, but today you have to have something different. Would you like waffles or eggs?*
>
> CHILD: *Toast!*
>
> PARENT: *Remember our rule. You can have choices, but you can't have the same food two days in a row. Do you want waffles or eggs?*

Then follow up the next day:

> PARENT: *Yesterday you said that you wanted toast for breakfast. I said you could have it tomorrow. Well, now it's tomorrow. Do you still want toast? Or would you like some yogurt?*

It's crucial to follow through on your promises—in this case, to offer the toast that the child wanted the day before. You've got to show that you're trustworthy. It's also crucial not to assume that the child still wants the toast. Watch out for the temptation to say, "What do you mean, you don't want toast? Yesterday, you *said* you wanted it!" Continue to offer choices and to step back from control struggles.

Often, this kind of dialogue will work. If it doesn't, and if your child refuses to eat, remember, it's not because she doesn't like the food you've offered. After all, you're serving only her favorites. Instead, see your child's refusal to eat as the control struggle coming to a head. Now's the time to remember the Eating Zones. Let your child refuse the food and comfort yourself with the knowledge that she won't starve. A snack is scheduled in a few hours.

But when children respond to any element of The Big Fix by screaming, throwing food, or having a tantrum, parents have to address the behavior. (Notice that the problem here isn't how your children feel about the food choices you're offering. It's how your children express their feelings that's the issue.) It's up to you how to address behavior problems, but it's important to communicate clearly both the problem and the consequence. You might say, "If you scream when I offer you your choices, I will ask you to stop. If you do not stop, you will have a time-out." Then follow through.

Spell out a positive alternative that your children can use to express disappointment, dissatisfaction, or any other feeling they may have: "If you do not want to choose between the two dishes I offer you, that is OK. I will choose for you. If you do not want to eat what I give you, that is also OK. You do not have to eat breakfast, but there will be no more food until snack. If you are upset, tell me how you feel, but no tantrums."

If your children frequently scream, throw food, or whine, it's even better to anticipate problems by talking ahead of time about what's allowed, what's not, and what will happen if they misbehave. Give them a friendly reminder before meals and snacks, to give them a chance to break out of their automatic patterns and develop better ones.

Finally, don't forget the power of praise! When your kids behave well at meals, reinforce their good work: "Thank you so much for eating the oatmeal this morning. I know you were hoping for a waffle instead. You can have a waffle tomorrow."

Disarm Your Little Baby-Bottle Bomber in Four Easy Steps

If you are introducing The Big Fix to very young children, fantastic! But it can be hard to teach older babies and young toddlers how to respond to food issues without tantrums. Bottle throwing is an especially sore subject for some parents. Here's a plan that lovingly teaches the lesson:

1. Pick up the first bottle bomb that gets launched, and while handing it back to your baby say, "When you throw your bottle I think you're done. Are you done?"
2. Your child will stare at you like you're crazy.
3. When the second bottle bomb gets launched, remove your child from the high chair or table and say, "OK, I guess you're done."
4a. If you think your child is still hungry, wait a few minutes and resume the meal. If a baby bottle gets launched, repeat the entire procedure, starting with step 1.
4b. If you think your child is no longer hungry, teach an alternative form of communication. End the meal and say, "When you are done with your bottle, put it over here"; "When you are done with your bottle, give it to Mommy"; or "When you are done with your bottle, say, 'All done.'"

Don't be surprised if you have to repeat this procedure three or more times during the first meal. It will take a while for your child to figure out what's going on and that you mean business. The key is to remind your child repeatedly what throwing bottle bombs signals to you, and what the consequences will be for him. You can tweak this strategy for all kinds of food behavior in little ones.

When kids challenge The Big Fix, it can be tempting to say, "Oh, my kids are just going through a difficult developmental phase," especially if you are an It's-Just-a-Phaser. Remember that it's also developmentally appropriate for small kids to push, grab, hit, bite, and scream, but most of us systematically teach our cute little barbarians to behave differently. That's what parents do—we teach. And it's never too early, or too late, to start.

THE BIG FIX FAQS

Q: *Do I have to implement Eating Zones before I implement the Rotation Rule?*

A: No. I'm giving you plenty of ideas for making The Big Fix work, but it's going to work best if you make it your own. Some families like to put the entire Big Fix into place at one time; others take it slower and introduce one new idea at a time. Others go *really* slowly; I know families who apply the Rotation Rule only at one mealtime, like lunch or breakfast. Some already have a version of Eating Zones at their house. They skip this part and go straight to the Rotation Rule. Trust your knowledge of how much change your family can tolerate at once, and you'll be fine.

Q: *Do I have to keep up The Big Fix for the rest of my children's lives?*

A: No. I suggest parents think of the first five years or so of their children's lives as a training period for good habits, but for some people that's too much. What really matters is that your children absorb the underlying lessons of The Big Fix. Once these new habits—of spacing out their meals and snacks and cycling through different foods—feel solid and normal to your kids, you can relax the rules a little.

Q: *Do I have to make sure my child eats only at the table during the Eating Zones? Sometimes we are in the car or on the playground during snack time.*

A: If you have a child who isn't particularly interested in sitting at the table, you should consider offering some meals and snacks on the go. Right now you have to balance two competing goals: teaching your children habits like sitting at the table and providing an environment that encourages young children to eat. It will not hurt your child if she occasionally eats in the stroller or in the car, if she has a picnic under the table, or if she eats from a tray in the living room.

Q: *If I follow the Rotation Rule, can I still use leftovers?*

A: Absolutely! I'm a big fan of leftovers. Anything that reduces the time I have to spend in the kitchen is OK with me.

There are several ways to use leftovers effectively within the Rotation Rule. The first is to freeze leftovers and pull them out sometime in the future. Or you can wait a day or two before using leftovers. Also, you can transform a leftover into a new dish by adding a new ingredient—for instance, by turning leftover chicken into chicken salad. Finally, if you absolutely must serve the same leftovers two days in a row, consider switching up the meal you serve it for (for example, use a dinner leftover for breakfast or vice versa).

The Rotation Rule is a guideline, meant to be used flexibly within your family system. If Grandma visits and prepares a special meal that everyone loves, then by all means serve it two days in a row. Just be careful that you don't use the special meal exception too frequently, especially if you have a child who gravitates toward being a rigid eater.

Q: *How different do foods in the rotation have to be?*

A: Ideally, you will rotate between foods that are really different: cereal one day, eggs the next. However, the point is to incorporate as much variation as possible while staying firmly within the foods your child already accepts. If you have a child with a limited diet, you can use a more subtle rotation.

If your child is particularly attached to yogurt for breakfast, you might offer different yogurt flavors, or even different brands of the same flavor. Other subtle rotations are sandwiches made with different kinds of bread, sandwiches cut into different shapes, different-colored pasta, hummus with carrot sticks one day and cucumber sticks the next.

Q: *I like to eat the same breakfast every day. How can I ask my children to rotate through different foods without being a hypocrite?*

A: It would be best if you rotated through different foods, too. It's not just that you would be modeling the right habits but that variety is healthy for you, too. However, you do not absolutely have to rotate. You do have to talk to your children, though, to tell them why they should rotate even when you don't. (Hint: For most parents, the answer has two parts. You are using the Rotation Rule to help your child learn to eat new foods; when he is more comfortable with a wider variety of foods, he won't have to follow the rule. Also, when your child grows up, he can choose to eat however he likes.)

Q: *Recently my son ended up eating pasta twice in one day because he had noodles at a friend's home and I had planned spaghetti for dinner. Did I just ruin everything?*

A: No. The Big Fix is a general structure. You need to stick to it as much as you can, but an occasional slipup won't hurt anything. Next time this happens, tell your son—with a twinkle in your eye—that he got a special treat but that tomorrow he's going back to the rotation.

Managing Mac 'n' Cheese and Other Kid Foods

Teaching Proportion

Now that you've got a strong structure in place, you're ready to teach the first habit: proportion. All this habit means is that you eat foods in proportion to how healthy they are. Pretty straightforward, right? Then why do so many of us flail with it?

The answer is that a nutrition mindset clouds up some of the most important aspects of the proportion habit. Clear away those clouds, and you'll see your way to teaching kids some lessons they can carry with them for life.

If you have a nutrition mindset, the main benefit of good proportion is that it directs kids toward foods with a specific nutrient profile. When you think this way, eating right is like making out a shopping list. You want your kids to pick up a little protein, consume some calcium, make sure they grab some fiber. But when you use a teaching approach, proportion is more like baking cookies. You're not as worried about one ingredient or another; you're thinking more about the overall blend. It's not enough to know which ingredients are called for, or even to get everything into the bowl. To produce the ideal mixture you need the correct amounts of flour, sugar, butter, and eggs *in relation to one another*. You've got to get the ratios right. The same goes for healthy eating; it's all about the relationships among the foods your kids eat. It means that they eat very healthy food more frequently than they eat mediocre food, and that they eat mediocre food more frequently than they eat junk.

It's true that parents with the nutrition mindset sometimes think about ratios. But when they do, it's a short-term kind of thinking. A parent with a nutrition mindset thinks about whether vegetables have crossed their kids' lips at any time in the last twenty-four hours and uses that knowledge to decide whether to make a big fuss about the kids eating broccoli at dinner. If the kids have recently eaten a bucket-load of candy or a mountain of pancakes, the parents try to get them to compensate accordingly. This is proportion, but on a scale that is too limited.

With the teaching approach, you think bigger and broader. The real question isn't whether your children have had any vegetables today or whether they've had candy before dinner. The real question is whether your children have the *overall* habit of eating more of all the truly healthy food and less of all the other stuff. Does the genuinely good grub—not the marginal, not the so-so, and not the only OK fare—dominate your kids' days? With the teaching approach, you're thinking about something else, too: whether the foods your children eat are shaping their taste preferences toward the healthy stuff. And with this approach you've got an eye on teaching them how to choose foods in healthy proportions even when you're not there to guide them.

THINK BIG

To leave the nutrition mindset behind, stop thinking about food in terms of individual items or nutrients. The key to getting pro-

Proportion vs. Balance

Sometimes people ask me why I don't use the word *balance* when I'm talking about proportion, as in "eat a balanced diet." My answer: because most people use the word to mean two things— both proportion *and* portion size. Those are two totally different concepts. Proportion is a big-ticket idea. It describes the decision to eat more or less of different foods according to how healthy they are. Portion size is more up close and personal. It applies to how much someone eats on any individual occasion.

These two concepts are related. Portion size often influences proportion—once you snarf down a gigantic plate of fries, there's rarely room for salad—but not always. It is possible to get portion size *wrong* and proportion *right*: You always eat gigantic portions, but you eat healthy foods more frequently than you eat junk. It's also possible to get portion size *right* and proportion *wrong*: You never eat more than you should, but you basically live on french fries. Neither of these configurations produces the long-term habits you are after. For your children to start eating the way you want them to, they need to learn how to get both proportion and portion size right. I'll discuss proportion in this chapter and move on to portion size in Chapter 8, when I talk about the habit of moderation.

portion right is to think big—to think about foods in broad categories.

Experts categorize food in lots of ways. You can think about whether a food is primarily a protein, a carbohydrate, or a fat. You can think about the meals or snacks a food is most closely associated with. You can categorize food by cuisine. None of these groupings helps parents encourage healthy eating habits.

The best-known method of categorizing foods is the USDA food groups: grains, vegetables, fruits, dairy, and protein. Their ideal proportions are depicted by the graphic MyPlate.

The MyPlate icon illustrates the principle of proportion really well. A single glance will show you how different food groups ought to fill your plate in relation to one another. Unfortunately, this way of conceptualizing proportion doesn't work so well for most parents. For one thing, even though it's a good goal to fill half our children's plates with fruits and vegetables, it's hardly realistic, especially if you have a child who barely takes a bite or two of anything green. That alone can make you want to give up . . . or turn you into a member of the Food Police.

For another thing, the MyPlate icon isn't in sync with how we eat. Except for foods like apples and oranges, most of the things we consume can't be categorized easily into one single group like "fruits" or "grains." Instead, we eat items that are prepared from multiple groups. Take pizza, which can contain grains, dairy, protein, and possibly vegetables, or even (in the case of Hawaiian pizza with pineapple) fruit. Do you know anyone who deconstructs a

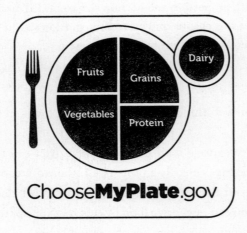

Out of Whack

In the absence of practical advice about how to implement proportion, it is not surprising that most kids' diets are out of whack. For instance, our kids get way more grains than they need. In fact, when researchers evaluate where kids get most of their calories, grains top the list. Add up all the bread, bagels, cereals, crackers, pretzels, granola bars, cookies, pasta, pizza, tacos, rice, popcorn, and other grain-stuff your kids load up on. Then compare this group to everything else your kids eat. See what I mean?

We live in a grain-saturated culture. You won't be surprised to learn that, on average, Americans consume more than twice the amount of *refined* grains than we should, because we hear that news all the time. Did you know, though, that to meet dietary guidelines, we would have to decrease our *total* grain intake by about 27 percent? That's a significant surplus!

Grains are not the only overloads out there. There are a lot of ways that our children's diets become misaligned, especially because kids naturally gravitate toward a repetitive style of eating. Some children I know eat cheese *constantly*. Others seem to subsist on milk alone. Most parents try to improve the ratios by throwing in a fruit here or a vegetable there, but that does little to correct the unevenness of their kids' overall diets.

When our children's diets are proportionally off-kilter, their other habits are affected, too. These kids gravitate toward the tastes and textures they prefer, they get used to the idea that they eat some foods but definitely not others, and they grow increasingly attached to a pattern of eating that includes fruits and vegetables only occasionally.

slice of pizza to see how proportion is playing out among those groups? Sure, some parents look at pizza and see dairy, especially if they are hoping to convince themselves that pizza is a good delivery vehicle for calcium, but no one I know dismantles their entrées to analyze how many grains, vegetables, and so on, their kids are consuming.

The final problem with MyPlate is that it doesn't reflect the way most parents think about proportion. When we're making decisions about what to offer our kids, most of us—no matter how much we know about nutrition—boil the process down to one question: Is it healthy or is it junky?

This question does a great job of pinpointing junk. But it does a lousy job when it comes to identifying healthy foods because of how the cutoff is determined:

First we detect and isolate the junk.

Then we label *everything else* as healthy.

This sets a high bar for designating the bad stuff—a food has to be *really* bad to qualify as bad—and a low bar for flagging the good stuff—anything that is even *kind of* healthy is considered good. In the end, we're left with a category called junk, which we can be pretty confident contains a bunch of nutritional trash, and a grouping we think of as completely healthy, which it really isn't.

Remember when I said that the nutrition mindset clouds your thinking about proportion? A problem with thinking of foods as either healthy or junky is that it misleads you into acting as if all the foods in the healthy category were equal when they're not. Some of the foods that get designated as healthy are truly optimal, but some are only average. Let's talk about pretzels, and you'll see what I mean.

Product	Calories	Fat	Sodium	Fiber	Protein
Lay's Classic potato chips	160	10 g	170 mg	1 g	2 g
Snyder's pretzel rods	120	1 g	290 mg	1 g	3 g

Pretzels seem like a healthy food because they are baked and have no fat. The status of pretzels as a food that is good for you is reinforced when people do what marketers hope they'll do: compare pretzels to potato chips, the ultimate junk food. I call this the Potato Chip Challenge, as if somehow surpassing the standard set by potato chips makes a food healthy. But does it?

Look at how Snyder's of Hanover pretzel rods stack up against Lay's Classic potato chips. Let's start tallying the wins. Ounce for ounce (about fifteen chips or three pretzel rods) the pretzels win on calories, fat, and protein; the potato chips win on sodium; and the two snacks are tied on fiber.

If you have a nutrition mindset, these numbers let you focus on a few nutrients and let you think that pretzels are a better choice. From a teaching standpoint, however, you can see the bigger picture. Have you heard about NuVal? It is a nutritional value scoring system developed by Dr. David Katz, at the Yale Griffin Prevention Research Center, and a dozen of the country's top minds in medical and nutrition science. The NuVal system calculates more than thirty nutrient and nutrition factors, ranking foods on a scale of 1 to 100, with 100 being top nutrition. What score do you think NuVal has given Lay's Classic potato chips and Snyder's of Hanover pretzel rods? It's 15. Both of them. (In contrast, blueberries score a cool 100.)

Of course, if you compare different brands you'll get different results. The overall pattern, though, will stay the same: Utz extra dark pretzels and Utz ripple potato chips both receive a NuVal score of 8.

I suppose you could look for a better pretzel, but this won't solve anything because there are chips out there that score better, too. Snyder's of Hanover organic whole wheat pretzel nibblers, for instance, get a NuVal score of 28. Baked Lay's original potato crisps are almost as good. They score a 25. But guess what? If you upgrade the chips again, suddenly they'll be ahead: Cape Cod 40 percent reduced fat potato chips score a 31.

Not everyone agrees with the NuVal rating system or even with the idea of scoring systems in general. Still, these scores are informative. By applying a uniform calculation to everything they analyze, NuVal makes it easy for us to compare the relative healthfulness of different products.

In this case, the NuVal scores illustrate my point. When it comes to salty snacks, you can look for the "best" choice, but nutritionally you're basically splitting hairs. The average NuVal score for the entire category of salty snacks is 15. If you have a nutrition mindset, you might end up focusing on what you want to see when you look at pretzels: less fat. But if you are using a teaching approach, minor nutritional differences become moot because you'll know that regularly eating *any kind* of salty snack produces the habit of eating salty snacks.

Pretzels: They're not clearly junk, but they're not truly healthy, either. There are more of these in-between foods than we like to think, largely due to growth in the processed-food industry. The health status of most of these items is difficult to determine. What would you say about Quaker breakfast cookies? Or about a Health Valley Organic multigrain double chocolate chip chewy granola bar? (It's low fat!) It's tough to know whether to put these into the healthy or junky category. The same goes for many of the foods that kids love: bagels, pizza, pasta, nuggets, and crackers. It's impossible to teach your kids proportion if you don't have a way to classify all of those not-junky-but-not-truly-healthy foods.

A BETTER WAY TO THINK ABOUT PROPORTION

Here's a clarifying alternative: Make a third category, one that contains all the middle-of-the-road foods. Now, instead of looking at a food and deciding whether it's healthy or junky, put foods into one of these three simple groups:

- **Growing Foods:** Foods that you *know* are fresh and healthy, such as apples, asparagus, and chicken. Eat these foods most frequently.

- **Fun Foods:** Foods that are sort of healthy, but you wouldn't call them junky, such as pretzels, sweetened yogurts, and chicken nuggets. Eat these foods less frequently.

- **Treat Foods:** Foods that you *know* are junk, such as cookies, french fries, ice cream, deep-fried mozzarella sticks, and cake. Eat these foods least frequently.

The best thing about this sorting system is that it tells you what to do about *everything* your kids eat: not just carrots, cantaloupe, chicken, and corn but granola bars and cupcakes, too. In fact, the real boon of using proportion as the foundation for teaching your kids to eat right is that it doesn't just help you get all those health-

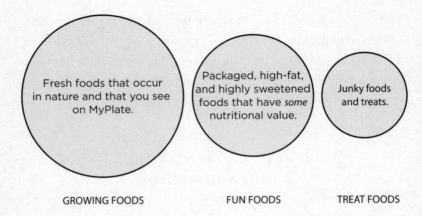

GROWING FOODS   FUN FOODS   TREAT FOODS

ful, nutrient-rich foods into their diets. It is a strategy for correctly packing it all in—the good, the bad, and sometimes even the ugly. And that's what eating right is all about.

This system is so clear that you can easily teach it to your kids. Even if they're too young to make good choices all on their own, you've got to teach them about the goal you're trying to reach and why. It's not called a teaching approach for nothing! If you don't teach your kids about what you're doing, how will they be able to cooperate with you? You can say, "We eat Growing Foods most of the time. They're the best for our bodies. We have Fun Foods less often, and Treat Foods only every now and then." This is an easy way to understand proportion, and it's one that kids can carry with them for the rest of their lives.

Are you wondering how to distinguish between a Growing Food and a Fun Food? Here's the good news: You don't have to start analyzing nutrition labels. This categorization scheme is not meant to be an exact science; it's supposed to be simple enough to apply to real life. Just step back and start generalizing. Think very healthy, sort of healthy, not healthy.

You can rely on your common sense and intuition to sort foods into the three categories, but I've provided an example of how a

Growing Foods (Fresh and Healthy)	Fun Foods (Not Junky but Not Fresh and Healthy)	Treat Foods (Foods You *Know* Are Junky)
Almost all fresh, frozen, and canned vegetables without a lot of added fat or sauces	Vegetables in rich or sweet sauces; oven-baked fries	Any vegetable fried in oil, such as french fries or hash browns
All fresh and frozen fruits; canned fruits packed in juice	Fruits canned in light syrup; 100 percent fruit juice	Fruits canned in heavy syrup
Chicken Fish Eggs Beans	Red meat Hot dogs Chicken nuggets Pizza Peanut butter and jelly	Fried chicken
Whole grain bread Brown rice Nuts Hot and cold unsweetened (or very lightly sweetened) whole grain breakfast cereals	Bagels Pasta White rice Tortillas Moderately sweetened breakfast cereals French toast, waffles, and pancakes Granola Goldfish crackers Popcorn Pretzels	Doughnuts, muffins, croissants, and sweet rolls Heavily sweetened breakfast cereals
Unsweetened milk and yogurt	Sweetened yogurt Chocolate milk Cheese, including cream cheese	Ice cream Frozen yogurt Soda and sports drinks

typical diet would be organized into Growing Foods, Fun Foods, and Treat Foods.

Parents who love this system will nevertheless have the urge to defend some of their kids' favorites. For example, what about cheese? Shouldn't cheese be considered a Growing Food, not a Fun Food? It's a point worth thinking about. Some middle-of-the-road items, like cheese, would be considered Growing Foods if not for a few problems. On the plus side, cheese is full of protein and calcium. On the negative side, cheese is loaded with sodium and saturated fat. Because public health officials recommend that everyone, especially children, cut back on their consumption of sodium and saturated fats and because cheese is now the single biggest source of saturated fat in the American diet, it is hard to make an argument that cheese is an *eat most frequently* food.

What about other foods? Shouldn't frozen yogurt be a Fun Food, not a Treat Food? After all, it's yogurt! And couldn't whole grain waffles be considered a Growing Food instead of a Fun Food? If you look around long enough, I'm sure you will find a nutrition plan that supports practically any position you want to take. For instance, because popcorn is a whole grain, many nutritionists think of it as a Growing Food. On the other hand, if it were salted, some nutritionists would place popcorn in with the Fun Foods, and if it were buttered, others would call it a Treat Food.

So why do I categorize popcorn as a Fun Food—besides the fact that if the nutrition world can't agree on the healthful status of something, it's obviously not *the healthiest*? Well, the classification system uses healthfulness only as a starting point; it is really designed to help you influence your kids' habits. Because your kids' eating habits are derived from their eating experiences, you want the foods you serve most frequently to taste like, look like, and *be like* the healthiest foods out there. There is nothing about the experience of eating popcorn that resembles the experience of eating any of the Growing Foods. To the contrary, the experience of eating popcorn mimics the experience of eating the other Fun Foods. From a habits perspective, then, popcorn has to be categorized as a Fun Food.

If you look closely at the three categories, you will notice that the Growing Foods are all more similar to one another, in terms of their taste, texture, aroma, and appearance, than they are to any of the Fun Foods. And the Fun Foods, as a group, are more similar to one another than they are to any of the Growing Foods. It's not that all Growing Foods are identical; they're not. Or that all Fun Foods are identical; they're not. But foods like crackers, waffles,

---

Save a (Small) Space for Treat Foods

I often say that what you eat isn't important; what's important is how often you eat it. There are people out there who disagree. They would say that your children have to avoid certain kinds of foods at all costs; anything containing high fructose corn syrup is one type that readily comes to mind. I think, though, that you can find a place in your children's diets for *anything* they want to eat (or anything you will allow them to eat). Candy? Doughnuts? French fries? I say, "Bring 'em on." Just keep them in their place. Not only are Treat Foods tasty, but they are *everywhere*. You can't avoid them. Your kids aren't going to live in a world without junk. If you don't teach kids how to put Treat Foods into their proper proportions now, you're sending them out into the world without an essential skill.

To limit struggles, consider asking your children to choose when they have their treats. "You can have one treat today. If you have ice cream after school, you'll have to pass up sweets tonight. What do you want to do?"

and nuggets have a similarity—they are basically the same color, offer basically the same crunch, and have basically the same flavor, which ties them together. The same can be said of other Fun Foods. Sweetened yogurt, applesauce, and chocolate milk, for instance, are all similarly sweet and creamy.

As you start classifying the foods that your family eats, ask yourself if there is a debate going on in the nutrition world about whether an item is healthy. If so, it's a Fun Food. Then check your instincts. If the item seems like a Growing Food—it crunches like a carrot or Mother Nature made it sweet—it's a Growing Food. If it seems like a Fun Food—it's processed crunchy or Day-Glo orange or it comes in a box, a bag, or a tube—it's a Fun Food, even if you think it might be healthful.

The classification system is not any more complicated than that.

FOOD FOODS: THE CATEGORY THAT REALLY COUNTS

Your kids' health depends on how well they eat Growing Foods. But *that* is a product of how well you manage Fun Foods. Overusing Fun Foods is like trying to fill a bathtub without a drain stopper: You never quite fill your kids with more of the really healthy stuff because the overall nutritional value of their diet is constantly being drained away.

Fun Foods are hard for parents to manage because they claim to be the perfect solution to our families' eating problems. We want to get nutrients into our kids, but they want to eat junk. Food manufacturers know this. They pump foods up with enough nutrients that they pass the parental sniff test yet are also tasty enough to appeal to kids. The resulting products land in the Fun Food category. It's not surprising that kids like these foods; they taste so

GROWING FOODS	FUN FOODS	TREAT FOODS
Least processed Least added sugar, salt, fat		Most processed Most added sugar, salt, fat

good. They're loaded with sugar, salt, and fat—three ingredients that are primarily responsible for the flavor, texture, and aroma of our favorite foods. These ingredients stimulate our appetites, too.

Think about how intensely sweet your child's favorite yogurt is. Ounce for ounce, sweetened yogurts have as much, if not more, sugar as soda. One 12-ounce can of soda has about 40 grams of sugar (depending on the brand), and one 6-ounce cup of sweetened yogurt can have 20 grams of sugar or more (again, depending on the brand). If your children enjoy YoKids Squeezers, get ready for a shock. Coca-Cola, which most parents forbid because it's so sweet, has about 3 grams of sugar per ounce; YoKids Squeezers have 4.5 grams per ounce.

Now, I'm not going to argue that sweetened yogurts are nutritionally equivalent to Coca-Cola. Of course the yogurt has more going for it. But close your eyes for a moment and imagine taking a sip of Coke. It's sweet, really sweet. Right? A YoKids Squeezer tastes even sweeter. If you have a nutrition mindset, you might try to convince yourself that the sweetness is OK because it comes from a combination of the yogurt itself, some "naturally milled organic sugar," and fruit concentrate. But if you are using a teaching approach, the question becomes, What does eating something so sweet do to your children's taste preferences?

The truth is that one sweet yogurt is no big deal, but most kids don't stop there. They eat sweet-flavored foods throughout the day. Look at the list of Fun Foods and you'll see that it is chock-full of sweet flavors, in the form of chocolate milk, fruit juice, cereal,

Is Your Child Learning to Love Salt?

The USDA recommends that children between the ages of one and three keep their daily sodium intake under 1,500 milligrams. Children between four and eight are advised to consume less than 1,900 milligrams of sodium per day. Look at how easily these numbers add up. Forget about the nutrition; think about how salty your kids' diets taste!

Kids' Food	Sodium
Breakfast: Nutri-Grain Eggo whole wheat waffle (1)	200 mg
Snack: Pepperidge Farm Goldfish crackers, Cheddar (11.5 oz. pouch)	360 mg
Lunch: Tyson chicken nuggets (2)	188 mg
Snack: Polly-O string cheese (1 stick)	190 mg
Dinner: Annie's organic shells and white Cheddar (1 cup)	570 mg
Total	1,508 mg

and granola bars. Pancakes and waffles are a double whammy—they're made with sugar and then served with syrup. Even sandwich bread tastes sweet. Add some peanut butter and jelly, and the experience is sweeter still.

Keep looking at the Fun Foods, and you'll see plenty of salt and fat in there, too. One reason kids love Goldfish crackers is that they're loaded with salt—as much, if not more, in fact, as many brands of chips. Chicken nuggets? Think salt and fat. Pasta with butter and Parmesan? More salt and fat. Pizza? Sugar, salt, and fat.

It's not an accident that sugar, salt, and fat are important features in the foods kids love. Food manufacturers have figured out the exact level at which people get the greatest pleasure from these ingredients. As I mentioned earlier, this is called the bliss point. Former U.S. Food and Drug Administration (FDA) commissioner Dr. David A. Kessler has written an entire book, *The End of Overeating*, packed with studies showing how eating these intensely pleasurable or hyperpalatable foods—those with just the right amount of sugar, salt, and fat—make us want to eat more of these foods; it's almost like we form an addiction. At the same time, these hyperpalatable foods make other kinds of foods seem disappointing.

Most children consume huge doses of hyperpalatable foods each and every day in the form of . . . you guessed it . . . child-friendly foods like mac 'n' cheese, bagels, and cereal bars. By one estimate:

- 70 percent of child-friendly foods have too much sugar.

- 23 percent of child-friendly foods have too much fat.

- 17 percent of child-friendly foods have too much salt.

It doesn't take long for children whose diets are filled with sugar, salt, and fat to develop what researchers call a *pervasive palate preference* for these intensely flavored foods. When they do, your trouble really begins, because children get locked into a self-perpetuating cycle of eating.

The more Fun Foods your kids eat, the more Fun Foods they crave.

Kids who get used to eating Fun Foods become less willing to eat natural foods, like vegetables.

If you've ever wondered why your kids used to eat vegetables but now don't, think about how many Fun Foods your children currently eat compared to back then. Infants don't eat a lot of Fun Foods (at least not compared to toddlers), so Growing Foods give them all the excitement their taste buds need. But after your kids get used to Fun Foods? Growing Foods just don't provide the same

More Sugar = Fewer Vegetables

Foods that are high in sugar, salt, and fat don't just orient your kids' preferences in a general, long-term way. They can also negatively influence what your children eat during the course of a single meal.

What do you think would happen if you offered your children a vegetable snack with water on one day, and the identical vegetable snack with Hawaiian Punch the next day? Do you think the kind of drink would influence how much of the vegetable snack your children would eat?

A pair of researchers from Oregon and Michigan decided to find out with a group of three- to five-year-olds, and guess what? The children ate a larger portion of vegetables on the water day. Not only that, the researchers noticed that even after consuming only a small amount of the sweetened drink, the children were relatively uninterested in eating vegetables.

flavor hit. Let me be clear: It's not feeding kids any single Fun Food *alone* that causes the problem. It's feeding children a disproportionate amount of the entire collection that destroys their eating habits. Flavor-hit foods train your kids to like corn chips instead of corn and to like strawberry ice cream but not strawberries. Flavor-hit foods never taste like broccoli, but they do taste like french fries. (Hmmm, maybe that is why french fries are the vegetable that toddlers most regularly consume.)

Fun Foods don't just move your kids away from Growing Foods. They actually move them *toward* Treat Foods. Yes, Fun Foods act like gateway drugs; once your kids get used to them, they open the door to more serious "substances." Remember the nutrition traps? Breakfast bars lead your kids to pastries. Crackers point them toward chips. And sugary cereal channels them toward cookies. If you have any doubts, try this experiment: Give your children a bowl of oatmeal, an oatmeal (or granola) breakfast bar, and an oatmeal cookie and ask them which two are most alike. Better yet, do this as a blind taste test. See what your children say.

The link between foods is so incredibly powerful that the only way to implement proper proportion in your kids' diets is to take advantage of the way those relationships work. This means giving your kids Growing Foods, not just because they're more nutritious (that's the added bonus) but because you want your children to *like* how Growing Foods taste. It also means limiting your kids' access to Fun Foods because you want to reduce their desire for Treat Foods.

By the way, this is the same reason that, from a habits perspective, a Treat Food can never be made more healthful. Oh sure, you can nutritionally perk up a cookie by making it nonfat and full of whole grain goodness and by eliminating the sugar, but you can't upgrade the way you classify it simply because you've upped the ingredients. To your kids, a cookie is a cookie is a cookie. Not only don't they care about how their cookies are made, but they're simply not sophisticated enough to figure this out. Whenever there is a classification conflict between habits and nutrition, habits must always win.

Put Proportion into Practice

Once you starting thinking about foods in terms of the three categories—Growing Foods, Fun Foods, and Treat Foods—the proportion habit is much easier to put into practice.

But what if your kids don't eat many Growing Foods? What if their diets are filled with Fun Foods? Don't worry. You can teach

Want Your Kids to Avoid Soda? Reduce the Juice.

While the American Academy of Pediatrics recommends that children one to six years old consume no more than 4 to 6 ounces of fruit juice per day, research shows that most two- to five-year-olds who drink 100 percent juice consume an average of *10 ounces* or more daily. Some public health experts recommend that children not be introduced to juice until after they enter school, so that they have time to develop the habit of drinking water and milk instead of juice.

Food manufacturers promote the idea that drinking juice is an easy way for kids to consume their fruit, but it is not. Juice has about the same sugar load as soda and none of the benefits of whole fruit. Maybe that is why, over time, children stop drinking juice and start drinking soda.

When researchers examined the top five sources of overall calories consumed by children aged two to eighteen years they discovered that at age two, milk and juice were the top sources of calories. By age four, milk had slipped to fourth place and juice had slipped out of the top five. By age nine, soda appeared as the fifth most significant source of calories. By age fourteen, soda was the single most significant source of calories in the diet.

Age Group, Years	#1 Source of Calories	#2 Source of Calories	#3 Source of Calories	#4 Source of Calories	#5 Source of Calories
2–3	Whole milk	100% fruit juice	Reduced-fat milk	Pasta	Grain desserts
4–8	Grain desserts	Yeast breads	Pasta	Reduced-fat milk	Pizza
9–13	Grain desserts	Pizza	Chicken	Yeast breads	Soda
14–18	Soda	Pizza	Grain desserts	Yeast breads	Chicken

your kids the good habit of proportion, but it's best to move slowly. If you've implemented The Big Fix, your family is already using the Rotation Rule, which means you aren't serving the same food (except milk) two days in row. At this point, your kids are getting used to a system that puts the parent in charge and that allows them reasonable choices. They're also adjusting to eating different flavors and textures from meal to meal and day to day, even if those differences are subtle.

To teach proportion, give the Rotation Rule a little tweak. Up until now, you've been rotating through the foods on your list without worrying too much about which foods are healthiest. That's fine—as I said, you've been getting your kids used to a *system*. But now it's time to take another look at your food list and note which of the items are Growing Foods. Shift what you serve so that those fresh, healthy foods are going through the rotation more often. At this point, you're still following the Rotation Rule, and you're still not serving any new foods or foods your kids don't like. But when you can, you're emphasizing the Growing Foods that they already prefer. You probably won't reach ideal proportions right away, but by exposing your kids *more* frequently to fresh foods and *less* frequently to fat, sugar, and salt, you are teaching their taste buds.

And what if there really aren't any Growing Foods on your child's list? Do the best you can. Serving canned peaches more frequently than crackers (even if the peaches are packed in a light syrup) will start your kids on the path to proper proportion. Remember, by reducing the number of flavor-hit foods your kids eat and by increasing the number of Growing Foods they in their diets, you retrain their taste buds in the direction of foods that are healthy for them. If you're one of the lucky parents whose kids are already eating a high proportion of Growing Foods, just keep the rotation going. By continuing to vary the taste and texture of the foods your kids eat, you'll make it easier for them to accept new foods down the road.

As you begin to shift toward more Growing Foods, remember the teaching approach! Talk to your children about the principle of proportion before you make any big changes to their diets. You can boil it down into a simple action statement: "We eat Growing Foods more frequently than Fun Foods, and we eat Fun Foods more frequently than Treat Foods." It doesn't take long for kids, even very young ones, to catch on.

Does the mere thought of asking your children to eat more Growing Foods make your shoulders tense up in anticipation of a hassle? Not to worry. There are plenty of easy ways to work more fresh foods into your child's day.

Serve Fruits or Vegetables at Every Meal or Snack

Don't think I've lost my mind, but plan to serve a fruit or vegetable at every meal and every snack every single day. This is one of the most effective strategies I know for reshaping your kids' daily diets. It's also the right lifelong habit.

Think about it this way: Even if your kids eat only a bite or two of fruit or a bite or two of vegetable five or six times a day, they'll take in a total of five to twelve bites over the course of the day. That meets or exceeds what most kids normally consume when the only time they eat vegetables is during dinner. The great thing about this plan is that even if your kids totally reject the dinner vegetable, you'll know they've already had a pretty healthy day. *That* will put less pressure on dinner, and when kids feel less pressure, they're more willing to eat their veggies.

Many parents shy away from frequent servings of fruits and vegetables because they don't think their children will eat them. But the reverse is also true: Kids can't eat what you don't serve. Because children are most willing to eat the kinds of foods they are most familiar with, the more frequently you serve fruits and vegetables, the more familiar these foods will become. Frequency is the anti-dote to fighting.

Serving fruits and vegetables throughout the day requires many parents to make a mental shift. You will have to stop thinking of *snack* as a type of food and start thinking of it as a time of day. Parents often ask me to recommend healthy snacks, especially portable ones. I always say, "Stop looking in the snack food aisle and start looking around the produce department." Carrots, snap peas, and green beans make great snacks. They come prewashed, precut, and ready to go. How about serving last night's broccoli? Or apples, bananas, and blueberries. Lemon juice stops the browning, plastic containers stop the bruising, and preprepping cuts down on the grab-and-go time. If you're in one of those situations in which you absolutely have to feed little kids in the car, you need to avoid choking hazards; you can offer pieces of soft fruits or lightly blanch some veggies in the microwave. Or take advantage of puree pouches. Although you shouldn't use pouches all the time—because you want kids to become familiar with the texture of fresh produce—they are brilliant for occasional backseat snacking.

Do you think it sounds boring to give your children fruits and vegetables this often? If you do, let me ask you this: Do you serve your kids crackers almost every day? Or bread? Or chocolate milk? Do you think *that* is boring? This is another mind shift you might have to tackle. Most of the children I know enjoy a wider repertoire of fruits and vegetables than their parents think. Count up the fresh fruit and vegetables your kids consume. Then add in the canned, the dried, and the pureed. Now mix this group into the rotation. My daughter loves snacking on frozen peas. Go figure.

Even if your children enjoy only a couple of different Growing Foods, you can still work toward a diet with better proportions. Remember the little girl from the last chapter, the one who ate only two different kinds of produce? Her mother made a slight adjustment to the Rotation Rule and put those two items—green beans and peach puree—on the menu every day. She also adjusted the way she served them, offering peach puree mixed with different things, just to get her daughter more accustomed to the idea of variety. You can do the same. Do your kids reject all fruits except apples? Fine. Put apples on the menu as often as you can. Just think about apples in a *bigger* way. There are green apples, red apples, plain apple slices, apples sprinkled with cinnamon, apples sprinkled with sugar, dried apples, applesauce, applesauce mixed with yogurt . . . you get the idea. Your kids won't get bored, and they will broaden their ideas about flavors and textures (a lesson that will come in handy when you teach variety).

Yes, I know that none of us will ever perfectly attain the goal of serving fruit or vegetable at every single eating opportunity. Some days you will be just too tired to slice up a cucumber. And every now and then you'll be at a playdate, and while there won't be a fruit or a vegetable in sight, there will be plenty of crackers. When this happens, let your kids eat the crackers. But setting the intention to offer your children fruits and vegetables *every time they eat* is a strategy that will serve you well, producing a net increase in your children's overall fruit and vegetable consumption.

Vegetables as Appetizers

An easy way to get more vegetables into the day is to serve them as an appetizer before lunch or dinner. This takes advantage of your children's natural hunger. After all, a lot of children don't deliberately avoid fruits and vegetables. They just end up inadvertently overlooking them. Here's what usually happens: You serve a meal with pasta and broccoli, and your kids gravitate toward the pasta because it is their preferred food. Then, because your kids are no longer terribly hungry, they pick at the other, healthier foods on

Goldfish from the Universe

One of the easiest ways to limit Fun Foods and Treat Foods is not to buy them. When my daughter was little, I decided not to keep Goldfish crackers or any other kind of salty, crunchy snack in the house because I wanted her to develop a habit of eating snacks like fruits, vegetables, and nuts instead. However, I allowed her to eat these items whenever they were offered up by the Universe (aka other parents, relatives, and schools). To ensure that we didn't become known as mooches, I made an extra effort to share our healthy snacks. There were a lot of benefits to this approach. I always got to be the good parent because I never had to deny my daughter's desires . . . outside of the house. And my daughter ate Fun Food snacks about the right amount of the time in relation to the healthy stuff.

their plate. But serve your children vegetables when there's nothing else to eat . . . and presto!

Two recent studies show that appetizers can dramatically increase vegetable consumption among preschoolers. In both studies, children aged three to five years were given vegetables before a main meal of pasta and cheese, steamed broccoli, unsweetened applesauce, and milk. In one study, the children were given vegetable soup first; in the other study, they were given raw carrots and dip. In the vegetable soup study, vegetable consumption jumped from one-sixth of a serving without the soup to almost a full serving with the soup. In the carrot study, the children's vegetable consumption increased from one-third of a serving to one full serving. And guess what else? The kids didn't eat less broccoli after consuming a veggie appetizer. The kids who were full consumed less pasta.

A Secret to More Fruit at Breakfast

One easy way to add fruit to your children's diets is to serve them unsweetened breakfast cereal. Recently, researchers randomly assigned children at three New England summer camps to eat either a high-sugar cereal or a low-sugar cereal. More than 50 percent of the children who ate Rice Krispies, Corn Flakes, or regular Cheerios put sliced strawberries or bananas on their cereal. In contrast, only 8 percent of the children who ate Froot Loops, Cocoa Pebbles, or Frosted Flakes added fruit to theirs. Don't think your kids will eat unsweetened cereal? Even though all the children in this study stated a general preference for sweetened cereals, everyone said they either liked or loved the cereal they ate.

Fruit for Dessert

Most parents dread dessert because it is the source of so much mealtime tension. Believe it or not, though, dessert is one of the most overlooked tools for teaching kids to eat right. You just have to change what you serve. Here's to fruit! Fresh fruit, canned fruit, fruit with a little sugar sprinkled on top . . . as long as it still looks and tastes like real fruit, it's a great choice.

The problem with most desserts isn't dessert, per se. Dessert is dangerous because it produces a bad family dynamic. The thought of dessert makes kids gloss over the good stuff to get to the *good* stuff, if you know what I mean. This, in turn, makes parents push the peas; do the two-more-bites tango; and otherwise beg, bribe, and cajole their kids into eating more of the main meal.

When you serve fruit, however, you preserve the pleasure of dessert—your kids will still enjoy it—but you eliminate the problems. Your kids won't clamor for a fruit dessert because kiwi just doesn't have the same appeal (or sway) as cake. Moreover, knowing that your kids can top off a poorly eaten meal with a healthy dessert means you can relax about whatever they don't eat for dinner.

And what about those times when you do serve a treat dessert? You won't be tempted to use the Dessert Deal because your kids will have already eaten plenty of peas, pears, peaches, and maybe even some parsnips!

Take some time to shift proportions so that your kids are eating more Growing Foods than anything else. As Growing Foods grace your kids' plates more often, they will naturally eat fewer Fun Foods and Treat Foods. They just won't have the room in their stomachs! And keep talking to your kids about proportion and what it means. Encourage them to think of Fun Foods as sharing time with Treat Foods. Offer a choice between one from each category: Let your children choose between crackers and chips, between sweetened yogurt and ice cream, between juice and cookies. As their palates become less accustomed to sugar, fat, and salt, their habits will change, too. At that point, you're ready to think about adding more variety. That's the topic we take up in the next chapter.

Laying the Foundation for Variety

Teaching Your Child *How* to Try New Foods

Variety is the second habit kids need to learn for a lifetime of healthy eating. It's no secret why; when children eat just a couple of foods, their diets are too limited. They miss vital nutrients as well as an amazing array of tasty foods!

If you're lucky enough to have a one-year-old who's still in the "I'll eat anything" phase of life, all I can say is take advantage of this time. Maximize the amount of variety you put into your baby's diet right now, and the payoff is going to be big. Very big. Variety early in life can dramatically reduce the effects of the neophobic, or picky, stage that most toddlers go through around the time they turn two. And if that's not a good enough reason to promote variety, think about this: The more flavors your infant gets used to now, the more flavors your child will enjoy throughout life. Two- to three-year-olds who eat a wide variety of foods are more likely to turn into adults who eat a wide variety of foods.

If, on the other hand, your child has already passed this small window of feeding splendor, you may wonder how you can make variety a habit in your house when your kids will use any tactic—

the lip lock, the head turn, the folded-arm posture, sulking—to avoid trying something new. Don't tear your hair out, and don't give up. In this chapter, I'm going to show you how to help your child get more comfortable with new foods.

If you've been following the Rotation Rule, you've already put the basic concept of variety into place: Your children now eat different foods on different days. This is an important first step for introducing new foods. Kids who are used to eating *different* foods are more open to eating *new* foods. Alternatively, kids who don't eat *different* foods usually won't try *new* foods.

Why? Because variety—even in the limited form of the Rotation Rule—teaches lessons that build on themselves. Variety shows kids that different foods need not be feared. It helps them discover and expand their taste preferences. When children get used to the idea that different foods are eaten on different days or at different times, they more willingly accept not having their favorites all the time. The *idea* of difference opens the door to new foods. In contrast, if you usually serve a predictable and unwavering menu, a new item will stand out as odd and strange. And yucky.

Some people find that introducing the Rotation Rule is all they need to do to get their children interested in eating a wider variety of foods. I think of this as the Rotation Rule Miracle. That happened to Gabriela. One week after she implemented the Rotation Rule, her extremely picky son started eating the kinds of foods most parents take for granted—turkey, fish sticks, chicken nuggets, bananas, apples, eggs, and rice—but that Gabriela had worried might remain off her son's plate forever. A month later, Gabriela told me that although her son was still a picky eater, he had continued to (cautiously) accept a wider range of foods. Gabriela was ecstatic.

If you didn't experience the miracle, don't worry. You *can* teach your kids to eat a much wider variety of foods; you just need to switch strategies. Stop trying to convince your kids to *eat* new foods. Teach them the habit of *tasting* new foods instead. Good tasters develop the confidence they need to go on to be good eaters. Think of this as a first-things-first approach to variety. In this chapter, I talk about tasting. In the next chapter, I talk about how to turn tasting into actual eating.

LOWER YOUR EXPECTATIONS

If you're having trouble introducing new foods, the problem may be that your expectations are too high. Like most parents, you probably tell your child that all you want is for her to *taste* the curried chicken you prepared for dinner, but deep down, you're secretly hoping she'll do more; you're hoping that she'll actually *eat* the curried chicken. Otherwise, you'll have to quickly jury-rig something else to put on your kid's plate or let her go hungry. Think of how much pressure that puts on the outcome of the new food experience. The stakes are simply too high.

When it comes to the task of teaching kids to enjoy new foods, pressure is your enemy. It makes mealtimes miserable. Parents push, kids resist, and everyone feels tense. Parents end up communicating disappointment and failure to their kids because it's hard to applaud that tentative taste when you're hoping for so much more. Kids end up thinking, "Why try?" On top of all that, the pressure creates a negative association with whatever food you're pushing. (It's hard to like fish when it's the source of so much family fighting.) No wonder many parents just give up.

You can turn things around. You just have to eliminate the pressure. Recent research from Switzerland shows that when kids feel like meals are enjoyable, they change how they eat. I'm not talking about the "draw some ketchup happy faces on your kid's plate" kind of fun and games. I'm just talking about garden-variety pleasure.

You know, when your family laughs and talks and enjoys one another's company.

The best way for parents to reduce the amount of pressure that children feel around new foods is to change goals. Stop trying to get your kids to *eat* new foods and start teaching them the habit of happily *tasting* new foods instead. Any foods. You don't have to stick to virtuous items like broccoli, spinach, tofu, and fish. Most kids enjoy tasting new flavors of ice cream, cookies, crackers, and candy. I know that these foods don't feel like legitimate sources of new tastes, but they are. Mixing all types of foods into the new food experience will change your children's attitude toward *new*. And that's the goal you're after.

The shift from eating to tasting may not seem like a novel strategy. Most parents think that's what they're doing when they say to their kids, "Just taste it, and if you don't like it, you don't have to eat it." But if you hear this statement from your child's perspective—"If you *do* like it, you *will* have to eat it"—it's easier to see why some kids balk. Especially if you introduce new foods the way most parents do, by putting a big heap on the plate at dinner. What if your child doesn't want to eat it, or even thinks he *might* not want to eat it? The safest course of action is to not even taste it.

The same result comes when parents tell kids, "Just take a bite, and if you don't like it, all you have to do is say 'No, thank you.'" True, many children will take a taste of something new when they are prompted this way, but they do so with the expectation of not liking it. In this way, the no-thank-you bite primes the pump for rejection—albeit a polite rejection—because children know that if they say *anything else* they'll be expected to eat whatever food they've just tasted.

Research tells us that kids need to taste a food several times before they'll accept it. That number is pretty high, usually somewhere between ten and fifteen tastings. When parents confuse tasting with eating, it's almost impossible to reach a number anywhere in this magic range. Most parents, even the ones who know that kids need many exposures to a food before they'll like it, give up after

Make "New" Work for You

Here's an idea: If you want your child to be more open to new foods, give him new experiences that have nothing at all to do with eating. Take him to a new playground or have him wear a new jacket.

Research shows the following:

- **Kids who are the most afraid of trying new foods are also reluctant to try new experiences.** Improve how your child handles "new" in general and you will improve how he handles new foods, too.
- **Fear of new foods isn't related to how much your kid actually likes something; it's related to how much he *expects* to like something.** Expectations rule the day. That's why exposing kids to lots of new experiences translates into their willingness to try new foods. It teaches them that "new" can be fun, exciting, and yes, even tasty.
- **Routine is important for kids.** Children thrive on knowing what to expect. But that doesn't mean things have to always stay the same. The routine kids need revolves around the shape of their day: the timing of meals, the behavior that's expected of them, and bedtime habits. New experiences fit nicely within this structure.

Put lots of "new" into your child's life, so that handling it becomes a habit, and your struggle to introduce new foods will be half over.

only a handful of tries, and I understand why. It's simply too frustrating to keep offering food to a child who's bound to reject it. I don't know anyone who wants to put the time and effort into making a meal only to have their child turn his nose up at it. Or who can stand throwing out food night after night. Or who can continually push their kids to eat something they swear they dislike.

When you change your goal from eating to tasting, however, all these problems disappear. Do you think the kids in those multiple-tasting studies are ever asked to *eat* anything? No way. In those studies, the researchers simply ask the children to take a single, solitary taste. That is what you've got to do. Then, cheer your child on because that taste represents success—and success is worth celebrating!

But many kids won't take even a taste of a new food. The secret is to make the process as safe and as unintimidating as possible. Begin by helping your kids predict what a new bite might taste like.

PREDICTIONS: TAKE THE SURPRISE OUT OF NEW FOODS

Ever put a new food on your child's plate, crossed your fingers, and hoped for the best? That's what Anna-Marie did when her husband, a superb chef, went a little wild with the ravioli one day. Instead of making the usual three-cheese variety that his family was accustomed to, Andrew made a gourmet ravioli filled with mushrooms and goat cheese. Then, instead of giving three-year-old Bryce a little taste, they plopped a plate full of ravioli down in front of him. "Shhh, don't say anything," Andrew said to Anna-Marie. "Let's just see what he does." Bryce took a big bite and promptly spit it right back out.

Anna-Marie and Andrew concluded that Bryce did not like the

ravioli, so they never gave it to him again. When I heard the story, however, I suspected there was a different explanation for Bryce's behavior. "What if Bryce was just surprised?" I asked Anna-Marie. "What if Bryce took a big bite expecting to taste the ravioli he was familiar with, and instead he got a mouthful of something else? Wouldn't that also explain Bryce's reaction?" Of course it would. Bryce was totally unprepared for the mouthful of food he was given, and nobody likes *that* kind of surprise.

In preparation for a workshop a few years ago, I put some applesauce into a clear jar. I added some food dye, so that the applesauce became a delightful shade of puke green. I added some chunks of fruit. Then I covered the jar.

When the workshop began, I held up the covered jar. I asked if anyone was willing to taste what was inside. No one was. Then I removed the paper covering so people could see the horrible-looking food. Only one woman said she was willing to taste it. She did, and said that it was pretty good. Everyone laughed, and finally other people said they would taste it, too.

There was a lesson behind this demonstration, and it was a big one: Being able to make predictions is key to trying new foods. It makes sense. No one wants to try a food completely blind, without any reliable cues as to what it will taste like.

Adults rarely have to taste things blind, because we have a large collection of food experiences to draw on. We're pretty good at sizing up a new food and guessing whether it will be sweet, sour, or spicy. Or whether the texture will be crunchy, smooth, or mushy. When we're totally at a loss for how something will taste, we ask.

But for kids, making accurate predictions isn't so easy. Putting something into your mouth when you have *absolutely no idea* what to expect takes a lot of guts, or a lot of blind faith, or both. Particularly if you've been tricked a couple of times, the way Bryce had been.

Research shows that children build up an idea of how an acceptable food should look and smell. Foods that are not sufficiently close to this idea are rejected, which explains why kids refuse so many foods before tasting them. Often it's because the food is a color they don't like or because it reminds them of something they wouldn't want to eat. One study reports a child describing a cauliflower as looking like a sheep. Would *you* want to eat a woolly sheep?

If children recognize a food and accept it visually and through smell, they will taste it. If the taste is acceptable, they will accept other foods that look and smell the same. If the taste is not acceptable, then foods with a similar look and smell will also be rejected. Sometimes kids can't even tell the difference between foods that look alike. For example, children commonly mix up cucumbers and zucchinis, two vegetables that are long, skinny, and green. As a consequence, kids use their feelings and experiences with one item (cucumbers) to shape their feelings and expectations about the other (zucchinis), but not because they think the foods are similar. They think the foods are the same.

What can you do to increase your child's willingness to try new foods? One strategy that *doesn't* work is to tell her it's good for her. The logic seems wrong, I know. Why wouldn't a child want to grow up big and strong? But research shows that the healthier children think something is, the less likely they are to want to consume it. What's the takeaway? The more parents threaten future health consequences ("You won't grow up to be tall," "You don't want to get sick, do you?"), the more reluctant kids will be to eat their veggies.

Why? Possibly because badgering kids about their health doesn't address their fears about new foods. This makes sense. You won't really care that a food will make you tall if you are afraid that it will taste like chicken lips. Researchers also speculate that kids choose foods for their hedonic value—how much pleasure a particular food brings them—so appealing to their logic just won't cut it.

Another strategy that doesn't work too well is trying to be an enthusiastic salesperson—"Yum, this tastes good. Want to try it?"—because it doesn't give your kids enough information. Imagine coming across Pantysgawn roasted vegetable pasta on a restaurant menu. When you ask the waiter what Pantysgawn is, instead of telling you that it is a mild, creamy goat cheese, he replies, "Yum, it's good!" How satisfied would you be with that explanation? And how likely would you be to order this dish?

Kids, like adults, benefit from being armed with information. You don't have to be elaborate (no need to recite each and every ingredient in a new dish), but you do have to connect a new food to something your child has already experienced. "This chicken tastes like the kind you eat at the Japanese restaurant because it has the same kind of teriyaki sauce." Even simple statements like "This is sweet" or "This is crunchy" are descriptions that can really ease the way for kids to try new foods.

Look at how little information it took to help Carlos, a seven-year-old picky eater, summon enough courage to taste a bagel. One day, when Carlos and his friends were each eating a soft, hot, salty pretzel, Carlos overheard one of his friends say, "This pretzel tastes kind of like a bagel." Carlos tucked that information away, and a few months later, Carlos told his mother he wanted to give bagels a try. And when he did, what did he say? "This bagel really does taste like a hot pretzel. Yum!"

UNLEASH YOUR CHILD'S INNER FOOD CRITIC

A great way to help your children become more comfortable tasters is to turn them into food critics. Present tiny samples of food for your children to test, and then invite them to tell you what they think. I love this strategy because it neatly removes the usual fear,

Food Games Build Food Acceptance

Kids build up food acceptance through repeated tastings but also through other, safer sensory experiences: seeing, touching, smelling, and even hearing. If your child is reluctant to taste a new food, let him play with his food instead. Consider a game of hot potato or what's in the box. How about encouraging your child to "paint" his plate with ranch dressing using a carrot stick "brush"? By letting your child warm up to a food in this way, you'll increase the chances that he will eventually be willing to try it. These games are particularly good for children with food sensitivities. You can find more ideas in the book I recommended in Chapter 1 called *Just Take a Bite: Easy, Effective Answers to Food Aversions and Eating Challenges!* by Lori Ernsperger and Tania Stegen-Hanson.

pressure, and control struggles that pop up when new foods appear. It teaches kids to make better predictions about food, gives them a more precise food vocabulary, and repeatedly but gently exposes them to new foods until the foods become friendly and familiar. And kids love to tell you what they think!

When I explain to parents that they can open children up to new foods by letting their child rate food, eyebrows go up. Parents ask whether this strategy will only harden their kid's bad food attitude. If they think asparagus is disgusting, why encourage them to express their revulsion? I understand these concerns, but rest assured that this approach actually helps nix a child's negativity.

Research backs me up. In a Louisiana State University study, a group of fourth and fifth graders were given cups containing samples of green bell peppers, tomatoes, carrots, and peas. Afterward, the researchers asked the children how much they liked each of the four vegetables. Over ten weeks, the children tasted each vegetable ten times. By the eighth or ninth tasting, the kids were much more likely to like what they tasted. There were a lot of ups and downs across the tastings, but the overall trend was toward liking the vegetables.

In another study, English scientists had a group of parents ask their young children to taste a vegetable they disliked (but didn't hate) for fourteen consecutive days. The children were given very small samples of the veggies. By the end of the two weeks, the kids showed a significant increase in how much they liked the vegetable. The researchers reported even more positive news: The kids said that the experience of testing and ranking a disliked vegetable was not torture, as you might expect, but fun. The experiment had also increased the children's willingness to try other foods. The only bad news is that some of the parents thought the exposure period was too long; 29 percent dropped out before the end of the fourteen days. The takeaway lesson is that you can change your child's taste buds if *you* are willing to expose them to small samples of foods over and over again.

READY, SET, TASTE

Transforming your child into a food critic isn't hard. Your efforts don't have to be systematic or scheduled. But, as always, you do have to talk to your child about what you're doing and why.

Talking to your kids is where the learning begins. Well before you ask your child to taste anything, have a simple conversation during which you talk about the importance of learning to try new foods. Don't worry that an open discussion will somehow derail the system. To the contrary, it will bring your child on board. After all, every day parents teach their children things they don't want to learn (brushing their teeth is one example that quickly comes to mind), and children accept the lessons. Give your child ample opportunity to express her feelings, fears, and concerns. Then problem-solve together. For instance, let's say your child is worried that you'll make her eat the food she's tasted. You can take this opportunity to reassure her: "I know in the past I've asked you to eat new foods. I'm sorry, and I won't do that anymore. I'll never make you eat anything you don't want to eat. Let's go into the kitchen, and I'll show you how small the tastes I'm going to give you will be."

This is a good time to stress that your only goal right now is to make your child comfortable tasting new foods. The more rigid or restricted your child's eating, the more you need to focus her attention on the big picture. "Remember when we went on vacation to Disney World last year and you had a hard time finding something to eat because nothing looked familiar? Even the chicken nuggets seemed different. Wouldn't it have been good if you were comfortable tasting new foods so you could have given those nuggets a little taste?"

Once you've paved the way with a conversation, the rest is easy. Just start looking for opportunities to have your child taste something new. Some parents like to have their kids taste a new food just before dinner, when the kids are looking forward to eating and the parents are already working in the kitchen. Others prefer times that do not carry a history of pressure and stress. Mornings, if they are not too rushed at your house, can be a great time for testing and rating. Or you can take advantage of opportunities as they arise— for instance, when you just happen to be eating something your kids have never tasted. No matter when you decide to offer tastes, aim to conduct taste tests frequently. It's not enough for the new food itself to become common. You want the *experience* of trying new foods to become familiar, too.

When you start selecting new foods for your child to taste, remember that you don't have to stick with vegetables and other healthy foods. Instead, stack the deck in your favor. Maybe start by taste-testing a new cookie. It'll get your child psyched for the tasting experience. Then if your child always eats mild Cheddar cheese, try selecting another cheese that is also mild and/or orange. As you progress, consider alternating between easy and hard tastes. If your son likes strawberry yogurt, let him try strawberry-vanilla or raspberry one day. The next day, branch out to a more exotic flavor and texture, like red bell pepper. The same approach works for children with sensory sensitivities. After your child is comfortable with tastings, start presenting slightly more challenging tastes. Don't move too quickly, though. Make sure you move at a pace your child can *easily* handle.

Because the goal is to make the experience safe for your wary child, you're going to have to think micro when it comes to the actual tasting. A single shred of cheese, one sunflower seed, or one-quarter of a pea are appropriate portions. (In the LSU study, the tomato sample was 1/32 of a medium tomato!) Don't be surprised if your child can't actually taste such a small morsel. Tiny bites make the experience even less intimidating. Next time she'll probably request a larger bite.

Ask your child to roll the food around in her mouth. Tell her she has your permission to spit out the food if she wants to. This is crucial. Tasting an unknown food is a risky proposition if swallowing is your only option, especially if you're not an adventurous eater or if you tasted something last Tuesday that was absolutely disgusting. Spitting instead of swallowing gives kids the courage to try. (Plus it prepares them to become wine connoisseurs when they grow up!) Have some napkins ready for spitting out the samples. Pour some water into a cup and explain that when adults eat a food they don't like, they drink something to get rid of the taste. Kids don't automatically know to do this.

Don't assume that if your child spits out the sample it means she absolutely hates what she's tasted. In the LSU study, 23 percent of the children spit out the carrots, but 31 percent of the carrot spitters said they *liked* the carrots. I guess they just didn't want to swallow them.

OFFER AN ALTERNATIVE TO "I DON'T LIKE IT"

As you start introducing new foods to your child, it's helpful to know that young kids don't have what researchers call *stable taste preferences*. When it comes to liking different foods, their taste preferences are all over the board. So don't take their comments too seriously. For instance, in one recent investigation, kids in England were asked to taste and rate the same five flavors of ice cream on two consecutive days. Researchers found that three- to four-year-olds typically rated the ice cream flavors differently on each of the two days. Kids five and up, however, were more consistent about what they liked. In other words, if your kids are younger than five, don't believe what they say about hating or even loving a food.

Even older children will change what they like and dislike with amazing speed, sometimes right in the middle of a mouthful. Some kids will like turkey on Sunday, claim not to like it on Monday, and like it again on Thursday. This kind of erratic behavior about food can make a parent want to give up. Try to see your child's fickle attitude as a blessing in disguise; it helps you understand that "I don't like it" doesn't carry the same meaning for kids as it does for adults. Chances are that if *you* say, "I don't like this food," you mean that you've tried it, possibly several times, and you find its texture or flavor objectionable. Most adults, even those with sophisticated palates, have a couple of foods they dislike. Bobby Flay, the chef, reportedly hates lentils. Ina Garten, aka the Barefoot Contessa, doesn't care for cilantro. You won't catch me near blue cheese. These are preferences acquired over years of thoughtful tasting and trying.

Resist the urge to ask your child if he likes what he tasted. "Do you like it?" encourages children to give food a definitive thumbs-up or thumbs-down assessment. Once something is labeled an "I don't like it" food, it's hard to get your child to taste that item again. And multiple tastings is your goal.

Instead, ask your child to describe what he sees, tastes, and experiences. This step has several benefits. First, it forces your child to stop and consider his food. Over time, this will break the habit of the knee-jerk "I don't like it" reaction.

Another benefit is that as your child learns to think more specifically about food, he'll become more comfortable predicting what different foods might taste like. He'll become more adept at distinguishing between foods (and less likely to reject zucchini just because it looks like yucky cucumber) and less frightened when something new hits his dinner plate. And the more precisely he can talk about food, the less likely he'll be to fall back on "I don't like it!" every time he feels wary of something new.

To elicit specific responses, try asking your child one or two of the following questions. Switch up the questions you ask from time to time, so that you hit all five senses.

QUESTIONS ABOUT TASTE

- Is the food salty, sweet, or spicy?

- Is it tart like a lemon?

- Does it taste like anything you've ever tasted before?

- Does the food have a strong or a mild flavor?

QUESTIONS ABOUT TEXTURE

- Is the food crunchy?

- Is it easy or difficult to chew?

- Does the food feel smooth or is it lumpy?

- Does it break into a million little pieces in your mouth?

- Does your mouth feel dry as you chew?

QUESTIONS ABOUT APPEARANCE

- What color is the food?

- Is the food bright or dark?

- Is it pretty or does it look weird?

- Does the way the food look remind you of something? What is it?

Two Hundred (or So) Tantalizing Words

One of my blog readers, Tricia, wanted her daughter to have an alternative to saying "Yuck" or "I don't like it" when she tasted a food. So Tricia developed a list of words to help her young daughter describe the foods she tasted. Now her daughter isn't just a great taster, she's got a great vocabulary, too!

- Temperature: chilly, cold, cool, hot, icy, lukewarm, refreshing, roasting, room temperature, scalding, smoldering, steaming, tepid, toasty, warm
- Taste: acidic, acrid, bitter, bittersweet, bland, briny, burned, buttery, chalky, charred, cheesy, chocolaty, citrusy, doughy,

earthy, eggy, fiery, fishy, flavorful, fresh, fried, fruity, gamey, garlicky, gingery, grassy, green, harsh, herbal, honeyed, infused, lemony, malty, meaty, mellow, mild, milky, minty, nutty, oily, oniony, peppery, pickled, plain, raw, refreshing, rich, ripe, roasted, robust, rotten, saccharine, salty, satisfying, sautéed, savory, seared, seasoned, sharp, smothered, sour, spicy, starchy, strong, sugary, sweet, sweet-and-sour, tangy, tart, tasteless, toasted, unflavored, unseasoned, vinegary, yeasty, zesty, zingy

- Texture: al dente, astringent, chewy, clumpy, crackly, creamy, crispy, crumbly, crunchy, crusty, doughy, drenched, dried out, dripping, dry, fatty, fine (small pieces), fizzy, flaky, flat, fleshy, fluffy, fried, gelatinous, glazed, gloppy, gooey, grainy, greasy, gritty, gummy, harsh, hearty, heavy, juicy, lean, light, limp, lumpy, lush, mashed, mellow, melting, mild, minced, moist, moldy, mouthwatering, mushy, overripe, pasty, powdery, rubbery, runny, satisfying, shattering, silky, slimy, smoky, smooth, soggy, soupy, spicy, spongy, stale, starchy, sticky, stiff, stringy, syrupy, tender, thick, toothsome
- Smell: aromatic, full-bodied, heady, odorless, overpowering, perfumed, pungent, rancid, strong

QUESTIONS ABOUT TEMPERATURE

- Does the food feel really hot or only kind of hot?

- Does the food feel like the same temperature as your mouth?

- Does the food feel cool or really cold?

QUESTIONS ABOUT AROMA

- Is the food very smelly, kind of smelly, or not at all smelly?

- Does the smell make you want to eat it?

- Does the smell make you think of other foods (like bakery smells make you think of bread and cookies)?

You may receive some over-the-top answers to your questions. (It tastes like badness! It smells like my sister's Diaper Genie!) Don't try to talk your child out of these answers. In fact, you should encourage a good giggle. It makes the experience of tasting new foods fun.

RATINGS CARDS

One thing you might want to do to make the tasting process more fun is help your child make ratings cards. I've provided an example below.

Then, after you've been through a question or two, ask your child to rate the food by circling the appropriate face. Be sure to meet your child's responses with neutrality. You may want to say, "Oh, come on! You love strawberry yogurt! How can you say that this new yogurt is really yucky when it's just regular old strawberry yogurt that is *also swirled with sweet, delicious vanilla*?" If you want to say something, try sharing how you experience the food. Don't talk about how much you like it. Instead, describe the sensory experience from your perspective.

One client encouraged her child to think of this as a science experiment. She created a journal with one page for each new food,

1	2	3	4	5
Really Yucky	Kind of Yucky	OK	Kind of Yummy	Really Yummy

with fourteen lines for each page—the number reflects how many times it takes most kids to taste a food before they feel good about it. My client encouraged her child to fill out the pages on her own. The journal pages looked a little like the one shown below.

If you try a journal, don't get hung up on making sure each page is filled from top to bottom. Instead, talk to your child about the need to taste and retaste foods. It's kind of like rereading a book. Every time you dip back in you get a new experience.

And what if your child doesn't want to keep a journal? It's no big deal. You don't have to keep track to be successful. The point

Food:	Broccoli	Food:	Asparagus
Rating:	Really yucky	Rating:	
Rating:	Really yucky	Rating:	
Rating:	OK	Rating:	
Rating:	Really yucky	Rating:	
Rating:	Really yucky	Rating:	
Rating:	OK	Rating:	
Rating:	OK	Rating:	
Rating:	Kind of yummy	Rating:	
Rating:	Kind of yucky	Rating:	
Rating:	Kind of yummy	Rating:	
Rating:	OK	Rating:	
Rating:	Really yummy	Rating:	
Rating:	Really yummy	Rating:	
Rating:	Really yucky	Rating:	

to the taste-and-rate approach isn't necessarily to score a win by getting kids to taste a particular food so many times they develop a liking for it. For now, the point is simply to help kids get comfortable with tasting new things.

FOR RELUCTANT TASTERS

What if your child insists that he won't do taste and rate? Don't take it too seriously, at least not at first. Children aren't always reliable reporters about what they will and will not try.

What do you think would happen if you presented a selection of fruits and vegetables to a group of kids ranging in age from five to fourteen years, asked them which items they were willing to try, and then two days later served them everything, even the offensive items? If you base your predictions on normal adult behavior, you would expect the kids to try the foods they had said they were willing to try and to avoid the foods they had said they weren't willing to try. It's surprising, but you would be wrong.

A recent study in Mississippi and Arkansas tried this procedure, and the researchers found some interesting results. Not only were the kids willing to try the fruits and vegetables they had said they would try, but they were also willing to try the ones they said they wouldn't.

But if it seems like your child really isn't ready to start tasting new foods, that's OK. The teaching approach requires a balancing act between respecting your child's decisions and forging ahead. One way to find this balance is to create a reward system.

You've probably heard that you should never reward eating, but sometimes that approach works. Here's an example: A group of two- to four-year-olds was given a tray of fruits and vegetables both at snack time and at lunchtime. The children were invited (not pressured) to eat either a fruit or a vegetable, and at snack time, the children who did were rewarded with a star. Fruit and veggie consumption increased. But something else happened. The researchers noticed that the children began eating more fruits and vegetables at lunchtime, even when they weren't being rewarded. Six months after the study ended, the children were no longer getting rewards at all, yet fruit and vegetable consumption was still up. The researchers concluded that the children came to find the flavors of the foods intrinsically rewarding, and as a result, the extrinsic rewards were no longer needed.

If you want to give rewards a try, consider a star chart. Each time your child tastes a new food he gets a star. (If your child is starting off slower, then give him a star each time he smells or touches a new food.) After he reaches an agreed-on number of stars, he wins a fun reward: a small toy, an extra book at bedtime, or a trip to the park. (Whatever you do, don't use food as the reward.) Price the rewards so they're easily attainable; it will keep your child motivated. For preschoolers, start by pricing rewards at one or two stars. Over time, you can make the rewards a little bigger and a little more "expensive."

Sometimes, though, even a star chart is too much. Some kids are simply more resistant to trying new foods than others, and not because they're trying to give their parents grief. Some children are highly sensitive to variations in taste, texture, or odor. (This makes them particularly vulnerable to problems with fruits and vegetables, which change as they become ripe and then overripe.) Other kids are shy or emotional or afraid of change. Any of these factors can make a child anxious about trying new foods. The more anxiety a child experiences, the more committed she'll be to avoiding that anxiety. This is especially true if eating, or even the thought of eating, produces enough anxiety that your child experiences nausea, gagging, and/or vomiting.

If you have a very sensitive and resistant child, you can still teach the skill of approaching new foods, but you need to go slowly. Tell your child that it's OK if she wants to start by touching or smelling new foods first. Follow the same basic procedure: touch and describe, or smell and rate. When she's at ease with this process—and if you've got a very sensitive child, it might take some time before you reach this point—you can move on to tasting.

If anxiety is a problem, teach your child to relax during tastings by using guided imagery. Talk to your child about how she can use what goes on inside her head to make trying new foods easier. Experts explain this as a form of "magical thinking" in which people use their minds to help them control worries or other symptoms, such as gagging. In one study published in *Clinical Child Psychology and Psychiatry*, the researchers recommend you help your child construct a story with images to help reduce or control symptoms. For instance, maybe your son's favorite animal is a horse. In the story, he could go on a fun adventure with the horse, galloping across fields. Suddenly, they could come upon a stream. Your son and the horse would then drink the magic water, and that would prevent him from gagging when he tastes a new food. Of course, you can substitute the horse for your son's favorite action hero or anything else he would enjoy thinking about. The key is to prompt your child to use magical thinking before each tasting to relax.

TASTING: THE FOUNDATION FOR THE VARIETY HABIT

This taste-and-rate approach is probably different from anything else you've ever tried, and it may seem like a lot of effort. But the more you expose your children to the sensory properties of food, the more comfortable they'll be when tasting new foods.

This strategy is effective. It can even work in tough cases, like three-year-old Adelene and her mother, Patricia. Adelene was happiest with french toast sticks for breakfast and meatballs for dinner, and she would often cry or run out of the room when a new food was served—even when the new food was bananas or something else that many kids find easy to like. In a bid to help Adelene become more open to tasting new foods, Patricia offered to take her to a restaurant, but then told her that she had to take a little taste of something new. Adelene agreed, and they went off to lunch.

At the restaurant, Adelene ordered meatballs, but they arrived covered in marinara sauce.

"I don't like that! I don't like that!" said Adelene. Her mother, too embarrassed to remind Adelene to find other words, went into a panic of meatball purification. When red sauce could no longer be detected, she offered a meatball to Adelene, who shook her head. It still didn't look or smell like any meatball she'd had at home. Then Patricia recalled the technique we'd discussed. She offered Adelene a teeny taste, and Adelene popped it into her mouth. If you have a seriously picky eater, you know how happy Patricia was at this moment.

Then that teeny taste came shooting right out. Patricia's shoulders sagged. She decided that the exercise had failed.

I, however, did a little victory dance when Patricia told me this story. She had done all the right things. She had asked Adelene to taste the new food (and not eat it). She offered the tiniest morsel so that the challenge wasn't overwhelming. She had allowed Adelene to spit out the bite she was tasting. Soon, I assured Patricia, her daughter would show more interest in new foods.

It happened in stages. Patricia continued to offer very small tastes of all kinds of foods—not just healthy foods but also treats like crackers and cookies. She asked Adelene a question or two about the food, resisting the urge to ask, "But do you *like* it?" Slowly,

Adelene became more confident with the tasting game. She was calmer when new foods were served because she knew she wouldn't have to eat any of them. Soon Adelene started looking at her mother's meals with interest. She asked to taste Patricia's sandwiches, salads, and once even went after a bite of fish. And one day, about a month after her first taste of the restaurant meatball, Adelene asked to taste a little bit of banana . . . and then ate the entire thing. She's still a cautious eater, but now she'll dig in to a much wider variety of foods.

I know it's hard to believe that your children will ever like new foods, but it happens. The more they get accustomed to a food, the more they like it. Even better, kids enjoy playing food critic. As they grow less fearful of trying new foods, they end up trying even *more* new foods. It's all about what kids are used to; it's all about their habits. And once your kids are used to tasting new foods, you can start showing them how to eat new foods, too. Keep reading to find out how.

From Pasta and Nuggets to Veggies and Fish

Teaching Variety as a Daily Habit

Believe it or not, you've already done almost everything that needs to be done to get your children ready to eat a wider range of foods. Using The Big Fix, you've put the right structure in place; you're not waging battles for control. Your kids come to the table ready to eat. They're used to eating different foods on different days. You've shifted their taste buds toward healthy foods and away from junk. And you've taught your kids to be comfortable *tasting* new foods. All you have to do now is start serving a wider variety of foods at meals and snacks.

Yup. It's that simple. You might think I'm joking, but I'm not. There are things you can do to transition your children from tasting new foods to eating them, and I give you plenty of strategies in this chapter, but basically, you've already done the hard work. Now you just need to start serving up the food. Any foods you like. Remember how you used to eat meals before the kids were born? And how gratifying you imagined family dinners would be? Well, that moment is finally here. You can start eating normally and stop being a short-order chef. You don't even have to keep track of which new foods appear on the menu. The idea isn't to put "Getting the Kids to Eat New Foods" on the family agenda. Rather, the idea is to start extending the Rotation Rule, no longer restricting it to familiar items, so eating a wider variety of foods becomes part of your kids' routine.

As you focus on teaching variety, keep proportion in mind. You don't want your efforts at increasing variety to upend the hard work you've done putting proportion into place. (What a waste that would be.) Moreover, it's by applying variety to proportion that you produce a proper diet. Think about it this way: You've already taught proportion by sorting foods into groups—Growing Foods, Fun Foods, and Treat Foods—according to how frequently they should be consumed. Now, if you teach your kids to cycle through a fairly broad range of items within each of the groups, you'll know they are getting the full range of nutrients they need. Green beans yesterday, broccoli today, and cauliflower tomorrow. Chicken yesterday, fish today, and hamburgers tomorrow. You get my point. Everything's got something different to offer.

Variety is great when it comes to Growing Foods, but variety at the low end of the nutritional spectrum is important, too. Cycling through Fun and Treat foods is a simple way to minimize the impact of any one "bad" nutrient on your kids' diets and on their taste buds. For instance, sugar is less likely to get hold of your children when they alternate among french fries one day, popcorn the following day, and candy the next day.

Variety and proportion are complementary principles. When you use proportion as the framework for promoting variety, any variety you establish creates the right proportion. It's a strategy that produces, and then reproduces, the right habits. That's why it's such a great system!

You're Never Too Young to Learn Variety

Did you know that you don't have to use the cautious "introduce one food at a time and wait two or three days before starting another food" approach that is recommended by American pediatricians? French parents feed their weaning babies a wide variety of foods from the get-go. One study documented French mothers making as many as twenty-seven changes in the kinds of vegetables they offered their babies (some as young as three months old) over the course of a single twenty-eight-day period.

Why? French parents are not primarily focused on identifying food allergies like we are. Instead, they're interested in promoting taste development. Because French parents have a different goal, they choose a different weaning strategy. The French method exposes babies to a varied diet, and teaches them to be comfortable tasting new foods. In comparison, our go-slow weaning practice means American parents can easily pinpoint which foods their children are allergic to, but they also end up teaching their toddlers to eat a monotonous diet and to be cautious of new foods. Doesn't that sound like most of the American toddlers you know? And the American method isn't any more successful at curtailing allergies than the French system: In both countries, the food allergy rate for children under five is around 5 percent.

So don't be afraid to introduce variety from the moment your children start weaning; it'll do them a world of good.

GROUND RULES

Putting new foods on the menu can seem like dangerous territory. What if your children refuse to eat the foods you serve? Seeing new foods on the table is probably scary for your kids, too. That's why you don't want to spring this change on them. Instead, help your children prepare for what's coming—and maximize your chances of success—by laying a few ground rules and providing some ways your children can opt out of eating something new.

As usual, start by talking to your kids. Tell them how proud you are of the work they've done to become great tasters and that now they're going to start seeing new foods at snacks and meals. Then reassure your children that you aren't going to make them eat anything they don't want. Remember the promise you made when you were teaching your kids to be tasters? Well, your kids do, too. It's important to reiterate that promise now. You don't want your kids to think you're not trustworthy. Plus, if your kids are scared that you're going to force new foods on them, they might retreat to their old "no tasting" position as a way of reestablishing their sense of security. Let your kids know that you hope they will decide (at least sometimes) to eat what you serve, but that it's entirely their own choice.

Next, reinforce your feeding structure. In particular, remind your children about the Eating Zones. Say, "It's OK to decide not to eat what's being served, but there won't be any food afterward until the next snack (or meal)." Then introduce some warmth and compassion: "I know it can be tough when snacks and meals change. So I'm going to do some things to make it easier for you."

Now tell your kids about some structured ways that they can reject what you serve. I'll describe these in a moment. First, I want to be clear about the value of these structured outs. One reason many children don't eat new foods is that they're never given enough time to stare questionable food in the face, to get comfortable with the idea of a food that looks, smells, and feels different. Instead, their energy gets sucked up by the back and forth that happens as parents try to convince them to eat, and they try to get out of eating. The struggle becomes a distraction, and the kids won't even consider eating what's been served. When you provide a strong structure and choices, however, the distraction goes away. You give your kids the time they need to come to terms with their issues and to summon the courage to eat whatever you're offering. It's how you help your kids grow.

The Safety Net: Always Serve at Least One Familiar Food

The first out you can give your kids is to provide a safety net food as part of the meal, something on the menu that your kids will eat. Of course, you can never be entirely sure what your kids will eat, especially if you're dealing with particularly tempestuous tykes. Just go with something your kids are *usually* willing to eat. This item could be rice or broccoli or chicken. It could be pasta or eggs or waffles. It doesn't matter what food you choose. What does matter, though, is that the safety net item is served to the whole family as a regular part of the meal. No special cooking. Not only does special cooking make more work for you (who needs that?), but it also sets the wrong expectation: "I don't expect you to like what I cooked, so I've already prepared something else for you." On the other hand, including an option that's easy for your kids to eat is just plain nice. Kudos for the cook!

Here's how this safety net might work at your house. Let's say you're planning to serve fish for dinner. You're not sure your child will eat the fish, so you also make plain rice and broccoli—two foods that your kid usually eats. When the family sits down, it turns out you're right. Your child refuses the fish. You shrug and say, "How about some rice and/or broccoli?"

There are a lot of ways you can work safety net foods into your meals. You can serve well-liked and familiar foods but offer new sauces on the side. If your kids like raw vegetables, put a selection of raw vegetables on the table for everyone to eat. If they like rolls, have some in a basket to pass around. Whatever you decide, remember this: The goal is to make a single meal that has at least one *reasonable* option for everyone. That means you'll probably have to identify a handful of safety net items that appeal to the largest number of family members. (You don't want to end up cooking a hundred side dishes.)

Also, it's important that you switch up your safety net item from meal to meal. You want to keep all the benefits of the Rotation Rule going. And don't resort to coaxing your child to eat the safety net food: "Well, you might not like fish, but I know you like rice. You like rice, right? Eat some rice!" Make a big fuss and you'll inflame the control struggle rather than extinguish it. Whether to eat is *always* your child's decision.

When you first explain this safety net to your child, keep it simple: "Don't worry. I'm going to introduce some new foods, but I will always make sure to serve something familiar." You can also talk about your goals here, one of which is to teach your kids how to cope with a less-than-loved meal without having a meltdown, throwing a temper tantrum, or running to the phone for takeout. When you think about it, I'm sure you can see that this is a pretty important life skill for kids to learn. I mean, most of us have to cope with consuming a clunker every now and then. And eating *only* rice for dinner never killed anyone. Your kids will need this skill if they're ever going to end up eating on a playdate, at a restaurant, or at Grandma's—wherever the food is guaranteed to be different and where they might need to make a meal out of just one or two items on the menu. Furthermore, as counterintuitive as it may seem, the pickier your child is, the more she needs to learn how to survive in "enemy" territory. So talk to your child about how to cope when confronted with foreign foods, and link this lesson to living in the real world.

The Backup

What can you do if your child refuses to eat anything you've offered, including the safety net food? You can take a hard-line approach and let the Eating Zones do the heavy lifting. Your child is free to reject everything in the meal, but he'll have to wait until the next Eating Zone before you'll provide more food. I have definitely recommended this approach to a number of families. However, many parents also benefit from using a second kind of out: the Backup.

The Backup is a single item that is *not* part of the meal but that your kids can elect to eat whenever they don't want what you're serving. When I introduce this idea to parents, many tell me they already use a Backup. In my experience, though, these parents use the Backup in a counterproductive way. The Backup appears magically, as if out of a hat, *after* the child rejects the main meal. It is chosen by negotiation:

CHILD: *I hate this dinner; I want pasta instead.*
PARENT: *You can't have pasta, but you can have a PB&J sandwich.*

In this circumstance, parents are using the Backup in a way that backfires. They let the Backup take the form of a preferred food (sweetened yogurt, cereal, and sandwiches are common choices), and they also let the Backup change from meal to meal. This way of using the Backup creates an incentive for kids to reject the main meal. After all, why challenge yourself to eat what's being served if there's always something more familiar and more tempting waiting in the wings, and if, when you get bored with one Backup, you can always choose another one?

A really effective Backup is different. It gives children control over what they eat, but it also encourages them to eat the food you serve. Moreover, because it is established as a firm part of the feeding structure from the beginning, there is *never* any negotiation. (That is a definite ground rule.) In this way, the Backup changes the way parents and kids interact at meals. There's no power struggle. There's no contention. There's not even any whining. The Backup is like a pressure valve; it releases enough tension that the system doesn't explode, but it doesn't release so much tension that it prevents the system from working in the first place.

There are five criteria for choosing your Backup:

- **The Backup must always be the same food item.** Pick *one* and only *one* food to use.

- **The Backup must always be available.** It needs to be on hand every time your child wants it.

- **The Backup must be nutritious.** That way you won't worry if (or should I say when?) your child chooses it every night for a week.

- **The Backup must be a *no-cook* item.** The point is to make your life easier, not harder.

- **The Backup must *not* be a preferred food.** You want your child to like but not love the Backup, so that there's no incentive for her to repeatedly choose it over the main meal.

There are a lot of foods you can use as the Backup. When my daughter was young, we used cottage cheese because my daughter liked it, but she didn't love it. I could buy it in small snack-size containers, so it stayed fresh for weeks in the refrigerator as long as it was unopened. Most important, though, cottage cheese is nutritious, but it's also extremely boring.

Over the years, I've worked with people who have chosen to use foods like tofu, hummus, canned beans, and plain yogurt as their Backup. Cottage cheese remains a favorite, though. (More children like cottage cheese than you might think, given its reputation as an awful diet food.) If this strategy sounds like something you want to employ, then talk to your kids about what Backup they might like to use. Explain the criteria and then brainstorm together. It's a great way to gain buy-in. Make sure the ground rules are clear: "You can choose to eat the Backup if you don't want to eat what's being served. But when the meal is over, it's over. If you don't want to eat the meal or the one Backup food that we've agreed on, you'll have to wait for the next Eating Zone to eat again."

It's pretty easy to see how the Backup works for kids. It gives them control over what they eat because they know exactly what their options are before they even get to the table; either they're going to eat something from the meal you've prepared or they are going to eat the Backup. What surprises most parents, though, is how the Backup makes mealtimes better for *them*. The Backup frees parents up to prepare the kinds of foods *they* like. (That's right, no more chicken nuggets for you!)

When Carol, one of my blog readers, learned about the Backup, she immediately proposed the idea to her five-year-old son, Jamal. "It can be your choice," Carol said. "If you don't like what I make for dinner, you can have some other food. Tell me whether you want that food to be plain cottage cheese, yogurt, or tofu. No more wailing and complaining. Deal?" Jamal agreed, and then chose cottage cheese as his Backup. With that, Carol started preparing the foods she and her husband liked to eat. The first night, Jamal started to fuss until Carol reminded him about the cottage cheese.

He immediately calmed down and asked for the Backup. Then, over the next few weeks, Jamal came to the table with his radar out. He would quickly scan the meal and politely request to have his cottage cheese. Every time this occurred, Carol quickly (and quite happily) complied. After a few weeks, though, Carol noticed that Jamal had started trying all sorts of foods: trout, burritos, tomatoes. You name it, Jamal tried it. A few months after that, Jamal stopped asking for cottage cheese altogether. What he didn't stop, though, was eating like a champ.

When I heard this story, I was really pleased, but I wasn't entirely surprised. I'd experienced the same transformation in my own home. Having a Backup gives children the freedom to try new foods because it gives them an out. The Backup also stops the drama and the discussion because the out is always "legal."

You can use the Backup for any meal, even those meals when you don't plan to dine together. Of course, it's hard to serve unfamiliar foods when you're cooking *only* for the kids. If your kids eat without you occasionally, don't worry about it. Serve what your kids like. But if the kids eat alone most of the time, I recommend you make an effort to put new foods on the menu fairly regularly. One easy way to do this is to use leftovers strategically. Whatever the adults eat today, the kids eat tomorrow.

WHAT FOOD SHOULD YOU SERVE?
BE AN OPTIMIST

When most parents think about introducing variety into their children's diets, they think of themselves as explorers, people whose job it is to *discover* what their children like. By now, though, you know that children's taste preferences are formed more than they're found. That's why I always recommend that parents think of themselves as

Are You a Parent Who Packs?

Ever been invited to someone's house for dinner and brought a separate meal for your kids? If so, you're a Parent Who Packs.

Believe me, I understand the rationale for always being ready with your own rations. It's better to be safe than sorry. When used as an occasional strategy to get through a strange situation—kept in your bag and used only when it becomes clear that your kids won't eat the host's food (what if it turns out your kids like chicken tandoori?)—then it's not a bad thing. But packing on a regular basis teaches kids that they should be able to eat their favorite foods every time they sit down to a meal.

Shift your goals from getting your kids fed to teaching them how to handle food-related social situations and a different solution emerges. Before you go out, talk to your children about what food will probably be on the menu. Then do the following:

- Let your kids eat before going out and then maybe again after you get home.
- Find something (anything) palatable from the menu being served.
- Encourage your kids to taste unfamiliar foods with no pressure to eat them.
- Insist that your kids always be polite.

You may be pleasantly surprised. Seeing others eat what they reject often provides just the right encouragement for kids to try new foods. But even if it doesn't, you'll have taught your kids how to be good dinner guests.

taste bud shapers. Taste bud shapers recognize that every bite of food influences their children's taste preferences.

Still, it's hard for parents not to go into explorer mode when it comes to variety, and I understand why. You want to maximize the probability that your child will eat what you serve. But that's a losing strategy. It turns out that parents are right only about half the time when they try to predict what their children will like or what they'll eat. Why? Kids are flaky.

Remember that ice cream study? When three- and four-year-olds were asked to taste and rate the same five flavors of ice cream on two consecutive days, they typically rated the ice cream flavors differently on each of the two days. Kids this young don't have stable taste preferences.

But even when kids are older, they're hardly consistent. A group of third through sixth graders in Germany was given two menus that each covered a week's worth of meals. One menu included their school's lunch options; the other had different options. (This ensured that the kids knew what some of the food tasted like, but not all of it.) The kids were asked, hypothetically, which meal from both menus they would want the most. Four months later, the students were asked to repeat the exercise. Only about half the students made the same choices on both occasions.

So if you can't predict what your kids will like or what they'll eat, then you shouldn't go searching for the perfect food. You also shouldn't limit mealtime selections to the foods that conform to your ideas about what your kids will eat. In both cases, you're just as likely to be wrong as to be right.

What you can do, though, is be optimistic. Get out those rose-tinted glasses and start assuming that your kids will eat whatever you give them. Of course, they won't like or eat everything you serve up, but that doesn't matter. When parents assume an optimistic outlook, they present their children with a wider variety of foods. Parents who adopt a more conservative outlook give their children fewer new foods. In the process, the conservative parents miss out on the chance to teach their kids valuable lessons about variety.

This is what Susie, a woman who attended one of my workshops, learned when she consciously switched from being a pessimist to being an optimist. Overnight, Susie said, her children became more adventurous eaters. Her five-year-old tried lobster, her two-year-old invented a smoothie, and both kids grew curious about carrots. Did they like everything they tasted? Not at all. (This might be a relief if your kids are tasting big-ticket items like lobster!) But Susie learned that the more foods she exposed her kids to, the more foods they learned to like.

A word of caution: It's tempting for parents to overuse a new food when they find something their children will eat, especially if their kids start begging for it. I'm thinking about what happens when parents move their children from regular Cheerios to Honey Nut Cheerios. When I ask parents to tell me how this happened in their families, they often say things like, "I thought Walter would like them." "It seemed like the regular Cheerios were getting boring." This is the right instinct: promote variety. What happens next, though, is counterproductive. Kids insist on the Honey Nut Cheerios instead of the regular ones, and when parents give in, variety goes out the window.

It's entirely normal to want to hang out with a new crush, but resist the urge to give in to your children's demands. Instead, work new loves into your kids' diets using the Rotation Rule. Repeatedly serving a newfound love might seem like it will seal the deal on that food, keeping it in your kids' repertoire forever, but it will undermine your broader goals. Being open to the concept of new foods is a mind shift for most kids. They need the *pattern* of change to reinforce the *habit* of variety.

Of course, it can be hard to be an optimist, especially if your kids have a history of refusing new foods. Although I'm confident that sticking to your structure is going to produce big changes for your family (especially now that your kids are confident tasters), I've also got some strategies parents can use to skew variety outcomes in their favor. Many of these encourage you to make very small changes, or even to take what feels like a step backward, as you keep the bigger goal in mind.

LINK NEW FOODS TO FAMILIAR FAVORITES!

I hope you've already been exposing your children to different tastes and textures through the Rotation Rule. Sometimes, though, parents tell me that they feed their children a varied diet, but as we talk about what their kids eat, a different picture emerges. One mother called her daughter's diet varied because she ate pancakes in the morning, yogurt for snack, and cereal with chocolate milk for lunch. This kind of diet is what I call the Variety Masquerade; you offer different foods through the day, but the items you provide are similar in taste, texture, or appearance. In this case, all the foods are very sweet.

To make sure you aren't falling for the Variety Masquerade, keep a log of what your children eat over the next several days. Look for patterns. Is your child eating a particular kind of food? Lots of cheese, for example, or foods that are smooth and creamy or foods that are beige? Note whether you are serving true variety or whether sameness has snuck in. Then tweak your Rotation Rule so that your children are exposed to different tastes and textures as frequently as possible.

But don't stop there. You can use your children's fondness for certain tastes and textures to introduce them to new foods. You do this by using a known texture or flavor from one food as a bridge to another food that you would like your child to eat. This bridge makes the new food feel less foreign. Remember how important it was to improve your children's power of prediction when you worked on tasting new foods? Well, that's how the bridge works; it helps your kids predict what the new food experience will be like.

You can start by using your kids' preference for sweet flavors to help pave the way to new foods. Yes, in this instance, sugar can be your friend! Researchers have long known that in rats, sugar can facilitate a long-term preference for certain flavors, even when the sugar is removed. To find out if the same holds true for children, researchers experimented with kids and grapefruit juice. A group of two- to five-year-olds in Florida was asked to drink and rate unsweetened grapefruit juice. About half the children liked the juice, and about half the children didn't. Then all the children were given sweetened grapefruit juice every day for twenty days. It's not surprising that many of the children who didn't like the unsweetened grapefruit juice said they liked the sweetened version. Finally, the children were given unsweetened juice again. Guess what happened. The group of kids who initially disliked the unsweetened grapefruit juice now liked it. To find out if the newfound preference for unsweetened juice would stick around, the researchers went back two weeks later. To their delight, it did: The group of kids who initially disliked unsweetened grapefruit juice still liked it.

It's unclear exactly why the sweetened juice taught the children to like the unsweetened juice. It may be that because the sugar doesn't completely mask the taste of the grapefruit, exposing kids to the sweetened juice still exposed them to the flavor of the grapefruit. It may also be that the sweetened juice helped the children develop the idea that they liked grapefruit juice. If so, that idea stayed with the kids over time.

In a variation of the grapefruit juice study, the same researchers found that serving sweetened broccoli and cauliflower (by dipping the veggies in a sugar/water solution) over three consecutive days was enough to increase how well college students rated these vegetables in their unsweetened form. So what's the takeaway? Taste preferences are more nurture than nature. And a little sugar can go a long way.

Here's another way you can use sweet flavors to build a bridge to new food. Parents tell me all the time that their child would never eat unsweetened yogurt, no matter the circumstances. "But what if," I usually ask, "you gave your child a bowl of plain yogurt and a bowl of chocolate chips? And what if you told her she could add as many chips as she wanted to the yogurt?" Of course, parents think their kids would go crazy, piling on a mountain of chips. And that's why parents think I'm crazy to suggest this technique. But this is what usually happens: The kids get excited, and they put a lot of chocolate chips into the yogurt. But they almost never pour in as many chocolate chips as their parents fear. Then they mix and mix some more, and then they eat!

Parents who are stuck in a nutrition mindset will see this strategy as a failure, especially if their child really does end up heaping a mound of chocolate chips over what now looks like a dab of yogurt. If you look at this from a teaching approach, though, you can see that what is happening is that your child is learning to accept the *idea* of unsweetened yogurt. And because the chips aren't perfectly blended into the yogurt, some spoonfuls will still taste more like the yogurt and less like the chips. And *that* will teach your kids what real yogurt—not the presweetened, preblended version sold in grocery stores—actually looks and tastes like. Furthermore, every time you let your child mix in some chips, the number of chips will inevitably vary, thereby varying the flavor of the snack. Over time, you can shift your child toward fewer chips by slowly downsizing the number of chips available for mixing.

Once you've created acceptance for plain yogurt with chips, then you can move on to sprinkles, maple syrup, or honey. Next, keep building that bridge by moving on to a mix-in that's a little more challenging. Maybe fruit jam. Then, as people of my generation used to say, "Keep on Truckin'." Consider adding fruit, chickpeas, cucumbers, or anything else your child might enjoy eating. Now you've got a healthy snack: plain yogurt with good-for-you mix-ins. You've also created a healthy variety habit by using plain yogurt as the base for different (sometimes sweet, sometimes not-so-sweet) concoctions.

You can use other preferred flavors and textures to build links to new foods. For instance, if your child likes crunchy foods, then look for new foods that are crunchy. Here's how it might work: Your child likes chicken nuggets, so one day you introduce fish sticks, pointing out that they have a similar kind of crunch. On another day you present fried cheese sticks, which are also crunchy, and so on. It doesn't matter that these foods aren't the healthiest. What matters is that they help teach your children to accept a wider variety of foods. After a while, you can bridge your path away from using child-friendly favorites on a regular basis. For example, you can move from chicken nuggets to fish sticks to breaded and baked fish and then to broiled fish. Of course, you can still allow your kids to eat their child-friendly favorites as occasional treats.

Alternatively, let's say your child likes chicken nuggets, but it's the chicken she likes more than the crunch. One day you might introduce broiled chicken nuggets, pointing out that the chicken inside the nuggets tastes the same. Then you might present your daughter with the broiled chicken nuggets and a teriyaki dipping sauce. After that you might move to broccoli with the same teriyaki dipping sauce. It won't be long before your daughter starts to notice

Don't Baby Your Babies: Let Them Take Their Lumps

Don't steer clear of challenging textures even if your baby seems to dislike them. When researchers gave a group of twelve-month-old babies steamed carrots that had been either pureed or chopped, all the babies preferred the pureed carrots, but some of the babies ate the chopped carrots, too. The researchers discovered that the babies who were willing to eat the chopped carrots had a history of eating complex textures, such as other chopped foods or mashes, at home. These babies also had more experience eating a wider variety of flavors.

If you worry about choking, you can do what these researchers did: Thoroughly cook vegetables before chopping, and make sure that the chopped pieces are about one quarter inch in size.

Still worried? Make textural changes slowly. Mix purees with mashes so they're half and half. Put teeny lumps into sauces.

The message is clear. Stop babying your babies. Instead, let them take their lumps. Textural variety is an important way that kids learn to eat a wider variety of foods.

similarities between old and new foods on her own. And that will help her be more comfortable accepting more variety into her diet.

HOW BRANDS BITE YOU IN THE BUTT!

Kraft Macaroni & Cheese. Annie's Cheddar Bunnies. Stonyfield YoBaby yogurt. We love our brands. They make feeding kids a snap, especially after you've found the products your kids will happily eat.

But for parents trying to teach their children to eat a variety of foods, the miracle of manufacturing—that food producers always turn out the exact same product (same taste, same texture, same look, same smell)—is also a curse. When brand names become an eating habit, some kids won't accept even small variations in the foods they eat.

Giving kids who are reluctant to eat new foods a Skippy peanut butter sandwich every day, because that's the brand they demand, is like begging your kids to never try anything new again. The more your children expect peanut butter to taste exactly the way—and only the way—Skippy makes its peanut butter, the less open they will be to foods that are different.

Does it matter if your children have one brand that they love? Not so much, if it's just one (although it might matter if they're starving some afternoon and you find the local grocer is out of their brand of peanut butter). But if you have children who eat chicken nuggets only if they are from Tyson, string cheese only if it's Polly-O, and waffles only if they are Van's organic, then the pattern is working against you.

If your children are attached to one brand of peanut butter, yogurt, waffles, or anything else, build some food bridges:

- Buy different colors, shapes, or flavors of the same brand.

- Buy different brands, but stick to the same color, shape, or flavor.

If your kids resist, don't try to coax or to convince. Reinforce Eating Zones with a safety net instead. The more comfortable your kids are with a variety of brands—with different amounts of salt, crunch, and other tastes and textures—the more comfortable they will be with variety in general.

What Not to Say at the Grocery Store

Experts tell parents that if they take their kids to the grocery store, the children will try new foods. But here's what usually happens: The child sees a new item and begs the parent to buy it. The parent, feeling dubious, asks, "Are you sure you'll eat it?" The child promises—and then is horrified when they arrive home and the parent serves the food. Everyone feels frustrated, and the child becomes even more set against the idea of "new."

Kids in this situation aren't being manipulative, really. Asking their parents to buy a new food is their way of saying, "I like participating in the grocery experience, and I want to be able to choose something, too." But they're not quite ready to commit to the *eating* part.

Instead of asking kids to pick out a new food and making them promise to eat it, let them participate in the shopping in other ways. Ask them to choose between two kinds of vegetables that you'd be willing to buy anyway. Use the experience of shopping together to talk about how different foods look, smell, and feel. If the store is giving out samples, encourage your kids to do a taste test. By keeping your expectations low, you eliminate the pressure that happens when you're home. And by using the grocery store as a laboratory of sensory experiences, you'll be helping your children become more comfortable with variety.

MAKE NEW FRUITS AND VEGETABLES TASTE GOOD

A number of years ago I ran into a woman in the town where I live who said excitedly, "I did what you said, and my daughters ate their vegetables!"

"Terrific," I replied, always happy that my advice works. "What did I say?"

"Make food taste good! So I sautéed the spinach in garlic and olive oil. My girls lapped it up."

Don't make new food dull; make it taste good. This may seem like the most obvious advice out there, but I can't tell you how often it's overlooked. This is especially true when the new foods are fruits and vegetables. Parents tend to rely on two methods: slice and serve, or steam and serve. When I ask parents why they do this, I get one of two answers. Either parents think their children prefer bland food, so they're reluctant to jazz up produce with a hearty dose of flavor, or they feel they've made so many compromises on the quality of the other food they serve—remember the nutrition traps?—that they don't want to "sully" the healthy ones. I understand this inclination, but healthy *boring* foods are up against stiff competition from all the other superflavored, junky stuff. This is a ratings war, and fruits and vegetables are clearly losing.

Like the mother who served her kids spinach, you can add flavor to vegetables using healthy additions like olive oil and garlic. For example, you can toss hunks of broccoli or cauliflower in olive oil, add some salt, and roast them in the oven to bring out their sweetness. But it's also OK to use preparation methods that are less than perfectly healthy. Add some cheese sauce to the broccoli. Cook carrots with a little brown sugar and butter. Sauté greens with bits of bacon. This idea goes for fruit, too. Try serving sliced peaches with sugar sprinkled on top, or bake apples and add some cream. These preparations may not be quite as healthy as raw or steamed, but they show kids that fruits and vegetables can be a pleasure to eat, not just a chore. They introduce kids to the textures and flavors of real produce. But remember the Rotation Rule. Keep mixing up the kinds of preparations you offer, and you'll teach kids a terrific lesson in variety.

There are times when truly unhealthy preparations of fruits and vegetables are still worth serving, just to get your child comfortable with a new food (and then as the occasional treat). In fact, some of the vegetable dishes you find in the market and at the local diner are ridiculously bad when it comes to nutrition, but they're fantastic vehicles for teaching kids to eat a variety of foods. I'm thinking about creamed spinach, for instance. Did you know that the creamed spinach at Boston Market has almost twice the fat as its macaroni and cheese? That's why it's so yummy. But don't fear creamed spinach or other inferior versions of new foods; once your kids develop a taste for the junky version of the food, you can use the bridging technique to lead them to a healthier preparation.

ALLOW FOR (SOME) FOOD JAGS

I'm pretty sure there is no research (yet) to back up the strategy my husband and I used to combat my young daughter's desire to eliminate foods from her diet, but it worked so well I've got to share it: We let her go on strike. My daughter would announce she was done with apples, and we would jokingly say, "Oh, so you're on strike against apples?" And she would proudly say yes.

Now, I'm sure she did not know what *on strike* meant. (After all, we weren't raising a little labor relations lawyer!) She quickly got the gist of the phrase, though. When my daughter was on strike, she didn't have to eat whatever food had suddenly offended her palate. We didn't urge. We didn't reason. We didn't discuss. We simply checked in and accepted. Of course, we also kept the offending item on the menu.

One day: Apples? On strike!

Another day: Oranges? On strike!

Another day: Potatoes? On strike!

One day I realized that the on-strike list had grown a bit too long. So the next time my daughter announced she was no longer eating something, management finally took a stand. "You can go on strike against only five foods," I said. "If you're going on strike against carrots, you'll have to bring something back."

My daughter considered. We waited. Times were tense. I worried. Would she accept my list of demands, or would there be a total work stoppage?

"OK, I'll start eating apples." And with that simple statement, a crisis was averted. Relations were normalized. A new contract was signed!

Food jags are a normal part of toddler life, and many experts advise parents to accommodate them. As you can see, I agree, but only partially. Without some limits, food jags can get out of control. That's because a child who uses food to express control is only temporarily satisfied when she wins control. That's right. She sits around feeling smug for about five seconds. Because that feeling doesn't last very long, the next time your child wants to grab some power, her only option is to do what she did the first time— eliminate another food.

The on-strike solution solves that problem by using a strong but compassionate structure. It allows some rebellion, but it sets some reasonable limits, all the while keeping things light. Of course, if my daughter hadn't accepted my limit of five on-strike items at any one time, I wouldn't have tried to make her eat the offending items. Instead, I would have simply relied on using Eating

Reading Food Lists Right

Food lists are one way that nutrition experts inadvertently encourage parents to feed their children a monotonous diet. If you're like most parents, when you come across a list with a title like "Ten of the Best Finger Foods for Toddlers" or "Top Ten Healthiest Foods to Feed Your Kids," you:

1. Scan the list.
2. Find a couple of foods that your kids will willingly eat.
3. Feed your kids these same foods every single day, confident that you're doing the right thing.

There are two problems with this approach:

- From a nutrition perspective, kids need variety.
- From a habits perspective, kids need variety.

So the next time you come across a list, use it as a gentle reminder of the different kinds of foods that your kids might enjoy. Work your way through the list and then go beyond it. For every item that is included, there are dozens that are omitted. Remember, by the time they're two, children don't need special foods. They can (and should) eat the same foods as adults. For very young children, there are only three exceptions to this rule: Meats and foods that are tough to swallow should be moistened (like in a stew), food should be cut into very small pieces to avoid choking, and foods should be prepared without very peppery or piquant flavors. But basil, garlic, lemon, and other strong tastes aren't just OK; they should be encouraged. Remember, variety really is the spice of life, even for kids.

Zones, a safety net, and the Backup to reinforce my feeding structure.

The on-strike solution is the same kind of fix I recommend for other kinds of food jags: when kids insist on eating sandwiches only with the crusts cut off, cucumbers only cut into squares, egg sandwiches only if Daddy cooks them, or only unbroken pretzels. Treat the demands as desires and accommodate them *sometimes*, but only when it's reasonable for you to do so.

BE HAPPY WITH A HAPPY BITE: HOW HIGH EXPECTATIONS UNDERCUT VARIETY

Years ago, a friend asked me if my daughter ate salad. The awe and admiration he expressed when I said yes turned sour, however, when I elaborated. "She eats a very small spoonful every night, and we serve her only items from the salad that she says she wants." In other words, back then we would lose the lettuce, but we would give her a few bites of tomato, cucumber, or another vegetable that was in our salad mix. We made sure to vary the salad ingredients from night to night as much as was feasible.

My friend responded with some version of, "I could get my son to eat salad, too if I did it that way. But that's not really eating salad." So he gave up trying.

Lots of parents feel this way. They want *more* from their kids— not just cucumbers but lettuce on the fork, not just one bite of salad in the stomach but a whole bowl. But I wanted to create a great salad-eating habit, and I knew that would take some time. For years we used what I called the Happy Bite: one or two bites—not a lot by most parents' standards, but bites that my daughter was happy about eating. And that's what we needed to cultivate a positive association with salad. Now my daughter regularly digs into an entire salad—lettuce and all.

Truthfully, though, there were nights when my daughter didn't want to eat even a single Happy Bite of salad. Because we serve salad as an appetizer every night, that's a lot of opportunity for fighting. But insisting that my daughter eat salad would have ruined my chances of turning her into a salad eater. Instead, we used her hunger to our advantage. We made sure there was no other food on the table until my husband and I finished our salads and we all moved on to the main course. (Think of this as a mini version of an Eating Zone.) Knowing that she would have to wait patiently for five minutes or more before getting to eat, all while *we* were digging in, usually provided my daughter with enough incentive to eat a little salad.

My salad strategy worked because we:

- Increased exposure by serving salad every day (but kept variety going by mixing up the ingredients).

- Eliminated competition by serving the salad when no other foods were available.

- Kept serving sizes small, so the challenge was doable.

- Stayed silent and allowed the structure to apply a small amount of subtle pressure.

USE RESTAURANTS THE RIGHT WAY

Bringing kids to restaurants is a potentially perilous endeavor. That's why it strikes fear into the hearts of many of the parents I know. Who wants to have their kids melt down in the middle of a crowded dining room? On the other hand, kids can learn a lot from eating in restaurants because they offer up fun, interesting, tasty, and unusual foods—dishes that most home chefs don't have the time, or maybe even the skills, to prepare. Just as important, restaurants are places where your kids can sample foods *you* hate. (Research shows that parents don't expose their children to foods they themselves don't particularly like.)

To use restaurants right, you must avoid the children's menu. With its standard choices of grilled cheese, hot dogs, and buttered noodles, the children's menu offers the opposite of variety. (Unless, that is, you never give your kids those foods at home.) I encourage parents to let their children experiment with the appetizer menu instead. It provides child-size portions of interesting foods. What's more, many appetizers are new, but not scary new. They're familiar, but slightly different: potato skins, dumplings, meatballs, quesadillas, nachos, and chicken wings. These might not be the most nutritious items on the menu, but we're going for variety here. (Besides, how healthy is the children's menu?) Other appetizers, however, are quite healthy and very appealing to kids: shrimp cocktail, chicken satay, bruschetta topped with tomatoes.

You don't even have to order your children their own meal. One way to use restaurants right to teach variety is to make a plate for your kids from whatever the adults have ordered. Let's say you've selected a chicken dish and your spouse has decided on a burger. Put a few bites of each of these entrees on a plate for your kids. Add a scoop of the rice or a handful of the fries and some of the side vegetable. You can even dole out bits of the garnish—it's usually some lettuce as well as a piece of tomato and cucumber—to make a little salad!

Sometimes, though, parents use restaurants to teach their children to be afraid of new foods. Here's a story to illustrate what I mean. One day I overheard a mother and her young child talking about what they were going to order when they got to the restaurant.

CHILD: *Onion soup!*
MOTHER: *Oh, you won't like that.*
[Long pause.]
CHILD: *Macaroni and cheese?*
MOTHER: *OK.*

Of course, this mother wasn't trying to teach her child to be a cautious eater. If I had to guess, I would say this mom was thinking that if she ordered the onion soup for her child it would go untouched, and she would have a hungry child on her hands.

I sympathize; I really do. But this mother missed an opportunity to expand her daughter's culinary horizons. She also contributed to the very problem so many parents complain about: Their kids won't try new foods.

So what could this mother have done differently? She could have honored her child's request for the onion soup after describing it to ensure that her daughter knew what onion soup is. Then this mother could have ordered something for herself that she knew her child would like, too. That way, if the child rejected her food, mom and daughter could have switched meals.

There's another kind of restaurant that parents can use to help expose their children to variety: the school cafeteria. You might be thinking yuck, but my experience tells me that many children enjoy school lunches. And they're not as unhealthy as you might think. In fact, school lunches are where children are most likely to be exposed to fruits, vegetables, and whole grains. Research shows that parents generally pack lunches that don't include these items and that are nutritionally inferior to what's served in the lunch line. Indeed, many home lunches include chips, prepackaged lunch meals, and junk food high in sugar. In one study of preschool centers in Texas, only 29 percent of the home-prepared lunches provided adequate servings of fruits and vegetables. And in another study of school versus home lunches that was conducted in Texas, more than half the home lunches included a high-fat or high-sugar snack. In contrast, fewer than 20 percent of the school lunches included these kinds of snack foods.

If you choose to let your child buy a school lunch, put some guidelines in place. One way you can reinforce variety is by allowing your child to choose a school lunch two times per week, sending a different home lunch on other days. If your child wants school lunch every day, don't fret. Many schools make variety easy for you: They don't serve the same meals from day to day. However, even if your child's school serves up the same monotonous menu of cheese-steaks and pizza, remind your child to use the Rotation Rule: No identical school lunches two days in a row. (You can also reinforce proportion by striking a deal with your child on how frequently he can have the sweets and treats. You could agree to chocolate milk once per week and plain milk on other days. Or french fries for lunch, but then no cookies for after-school snack.)

On the other hand, I'm not knocking unhealthy home lunches. In fact, I often tell parents that sending a *different* unhealthy lunch every day that your children will eat is a better strategy than sending the *same* healthy lunch every day you know your kids will eat. Remember, we're teaching the habit of variety, and learning good habits will ultimately lead to good nutrition. As your children's habits improve, you will be able to improve the quality of the lunches you pack. Also, an ever-changing unhealthy lunch that kids will eat is also better than a healthy lunch that kids discard. Not just because you want your kids to have enough sustenance to get through the day. Sending a lunch full of healthy food that your kids dislike reinforces the seek-and-destroy habit: Kids seek out, then destroy, the food they *know* they won't eat. I know this is controversial advice, but promoting the long-term habit of variety is a strategy that will pay off nutritionally as your children learn to eat better.

Variety takes a little time to cultivate. For some kids, it takes more than a little time. But have faith! Parents with the teaching mindset don't focus on getting their kids to eat a new food right away; they are patient as kids acquaint themselves with the idea of a new flavor, smell, or texture. These parents are willing to let their kids bridge slowly from one food to another, and they let their kids try some less-than-healthy foods so that their kids make a positive association with "new."

If your child takes months before she eats something new, don't worry. It will happen. Some kids will always be cautious around new foods, but every child can increase her comfort level with the idea of "new." And even young children can master the principle behind variety. Three-year-old Hector proved this point when he recently told his mother, "Those pancakes Granny made were yummy. I want to have them another day." "Another day?" his mother queried. "Yes. Another day," Hector said. "Not today, 'cause we need to eat a va-why-ittee of food."

B. Should you override what your kids say about their hunger and tell them they need to eat more?

If you're like most parents, you know the answer is A, but you act as if the answer were B. I get it. Letting kids dictate how much they eat is a great goal. Every parent knows, though, that it doesn't always cut the mustard in the real world, where children have hunger-induced meltdowns and a lot of kids would rather play than eat. Maybe that's why parents don't tend to even ask their little ones if they're full. What happens when parents do ask? When children say they're full, their parents ignore them. Do any of these reactions sound familiar?

Disbelief. But you've only had a few bites. You can't be full.

Encouragement. You can do it; finish a few more bites.

Pleading. Please just eat this much and you're done.

Bribing. There are cookies waiting when you finish up.

The Hunger Dilemma presents itself on the flipside, too. Should you believe your kids when they say they're starving? (Is it possible that a five-year-old absolutely needs two huge helpings of pasta? Or that a first grader needs three after-school snacks?) Or should you regulate how much your kids eat? From this angle, the questions are just as challenging. But as you'll see in this chapter, you can teach kids how to get moderation right.

How We Teach Kids to Overeat (or Undereat)

Parents have good reason to distrust that their children will get portion size right. Young children often have difficulty matching the words *hungry* and *full* with their feelings. Haven't you ever noticed that children sometimes say they are hungry but then they don't eat? When my daughter was little, she often said her tummy hurt. Sometimes that meant she was hungry; sometimes it meant she was sick. I had to use detective skills to determine the right course of action: Should I feed her or call the doctor?

On the other hand, there's no denying that sometimes children deliberately misrepresent the state of their stomachs. Are you serving a dinner your kids don't like? They're full. Are there cookies for dessert? They're hungry. It's enough to drive you crazy.

Still, here's the truth: *Even though there are plenty of reasons not to trust what your children say about being hungry or full, you really have no other options. How much your children eat is something they have to decide for themselves.* Your kids have to be their own eating experts because it is impossible for parents (or even for pediatricians) to know how much children need to eat at any given time. Energy needs depend on so many things: how much children are growing, how active they have been that day, how filling the previous meal was, whether they're feeling sick.

Even if it turns out, by some stroke of magic, that you *do* know how much your kids ought to eat, you still shouldn't interfere. Teaching your kids to trust *your* instincts rather than their own instincts prevents your children from learning how to self-regulate. They don't learn to pace themselves so that they have room for vegetables *and* for dessert; they don't learn to stop eating until they finish the entire bag of chips; and they don't learn how to get through holidays like Halloween without, shall we say, heaving. Moreover, your doubt produces a self-fulfilling prophecy: You don't think your children can self-regulate, so you interfere. Because you interfere, your kids never learn to self-regulate.

When parents pressure children to eat more food than they want—"If you don't eat all your food, you won't get dessert"; "You haven't eaten enough; take two more bites"; "Finish your food; there are starving kids in India!"—kids learn to ignore their internal cues of hunger and fullness. Instead, they start looking for external cues, like parental approval and whether they've eaten their entire portions.

The path from pleasing parents to overeating is fairly straightforward: You ask your kids to eat more food, and they do (especially if they're trying to "earn" dessert). Portion size is another, subtler, way parents unintentionally teach kids to overeat. There is incontrovertible evidence that the bigger the serving size, the more people consume, whether they intend to or not. This goes for kids, too. If you double the amount of food you put on your children's plates, they'll eat about 25 percent more food. And guess what? They'll eat this much more *regardless of how hungry they are*.

You've probably heard that children instinctively know how much to eat, but actually, the link between body and brain is easily disrupted early in life. A lot of kids are already ignoring their internal hunger and fullness cues by the age of three. And when your kids get used to eating larger portions—either because you ask them to eat a few more bites or because you serve more food than your kids need—you set in motion a lifelong habit. It turns out that people try to eat the same visual amount of food from meal to meal, regardless of how hungry they are. It's called our consumption norm. That might not be so bad if portions were reasonably sized, but outsize portions now dominate the landscape.

I'm sure you don't need to be convinced that portion sizes have exploded, but look at this trend. Brian Wansink and his colleagues at Cornell report that some entrées in the 2006 edition of the *Joy of Cooking*, for instance, yield servings that are as much as 62 percent larger than the identical recipe from the original 1920 edition. Dietician Lisa Young has shown that the chocolate chip cookie recipe on the back of the Nestlé Toll House semisweet chocolate morsels bag went from making one hundred cookies to making only sixty cookies. The ingredient amounts are the same; it's the cookies that have grown bigger. At the same time, popular foods, like bagels, have also exploded in size. In the 1960s, bagels weighed around 2 ounces; in 2000, they weighed between 4 and 6 ounces. The evidence goes on.

If you're parenting an undereater or a child with a slight appetite, you might feel conflicted right about now. You might be willing to risk teaching your kids to overeat—it seems like such an unlikely outcome—to make sure your kids don't undereat. Well, I've got news for you: If you resort to pressuring your undereating child to eat more than she wants, your efforts will be counterproductive. Undereaters don't respond to pressure the way typical eaters do. In the face of pressure, many undereaters eat less food *regardless of how hungry they are*. It's how they exert a measure of control over their lives.

Imagine the scenario: You have a child who isn't terribly interested in eating. You nudge, cajole, and try to tempt, but your child refuses to budge. What do you do? Naturally, you intensify your efforts. You offer more tempting food, like ice cream! You make some idle threats. ("If you don't eat something, we aren't going to the park.") You offer food at any, and every, opportunity. Still, your efforts go nowhere. So what do you do? Try even harder. But that makes the situation even worse. Now you're in the middle of a full-fledged control struggle, and anything you do to out-control your child will backfire. It's not just a short-term problem, either. In the long run, pressure produces the same ill effect in undereaters as it does in all children: It makes them less sensitive to their own hunger and fullness cues.

Almost anything parents do to control how much their children eat will ultimately lead to out-of-whack eating. If you pressure your kids to eat less—"You've had enough now, you need to stop"—your kids will probably eat as much as they can whenever they get the chance, even if they're not particularly hungry. This is especially true if you've been overrestrictive in regard to sweets and treats. (I'm sure you've met kids who hoard M&M's during playdates, at parties, and at Grandma's house.)

If you push your children to eat more when what you are really trying to do is get them to eat differently, you'll also teach your kids to overeat. When parents use the Dessert Deal ("eat your broccoli if you want a brownie"), they risk teaching their children that it is normal to eat dessert when they're *already* full. It's healthier for them to learn how to save room for dessert.

The Dessert Deal backfires in another way, too. It may work in the short term, but in the long term, pressure loses its effectiveness. And by increasing the desirability of dessert and decreasing the desirability of vegetables, parents get stuck in another vicious circle: Kids don't eat their veggies, parents push, kids eat fewer veggies. More pushing doesn't just make mealtimes miserable, it also leads to more external eating.

So what can you do? This is the time for the big-picture teaching approach. Start by reinforcing your kids' internal hunger and fullness cues. It is the only way your kids will learn to manage moderation on their own. (You do want them to move out one day, don't you?) Then teach them how to navigate the abundant world they live in. Will they make mistakes? Sure, but that's not a problem if you turn those mistakes into teaching moments. I'm going to show you how. Let's get started.

Eat Every Bite: A Lesson That Lingers

The Clean Plate Club has a lot of members. Recently, researchers at the University of Bristol, UK, wanted to find out how frequently plate cleaning occurs. They surveyed more than seven hundred adults and discovered that people are more likely to finish their food than to eat to satisfy their hunger:

- 91 percent said they had eaten every bite of their last meal.
- 28 percent finished their food even though they had been full.
- 86 percent said they had planned to consume the entire meal even before they sat down to eat.
- 7 percent ate less than they had planned.

Where do adults learn to clean their plates? The answer: in childhood.

RESOLVE THE HUNGER DILEMMA

The most widely recommended solution to the Hunger Dilemma is called the Division of Responsibility. Developed by dietician Ellyn Satter, the Division of Responsibility says that parents decide what, when, and where food is served, and children decide how much, and which, of these foods they want to eat.

The thing I love about the Division of Responsibility is that it is an excellent model of shared control. Parents provide lots of healthy food at regularly scheduled meals and snacks (which I hope you recognize as a combination of Eating Zones and the principles of variety and proportion). Then parents let their children get down to the business of figuring out how much food they want to eat. There's no stress, there's no fighting, and there's no pressure. Sounds good, right? Especially because you probably don't just want to nourish your kids but also want everyone to enjoy family meals.

What I don't love about the Division of Responsibility is that it is too passive. It doesn't teach children; it leaves kids to figure things out *on their own*. Not only do many children need support to tap into their own hunger and satiation cues accurately, but it is almost impossible for most of the parents I know to sit back silently while they watch their children bypass the broccoli *yet again*. Then parents end up pushing the vegetables or bribing with dessert. They're doing the things that prevent kids from learning to self-regulate.

Fortunately, you can teach your children the principle of moderation without any unintended consequences as long as you integrate your teaching into a strong structure. Remember, strong structure = less pressure. Let's start by improving how well your children tune into their internal cues.

HELP KIDS IDENTIFY WHEN THEY'RE HUNGRY AND WHEN THEY'RE FULL

Our bodies send us cues to let us know when we're hungry and when we're full. But many children don't know how to hear these cues. Here's a cool way that researchers in Colorado taught a group of three- and four-year-olds to self-regulate their eating that you can try at home. It is easy and fun.

First, talk to your children about the concepts of hunger, fullness, and overeating, and how these body states feel. You might want to use an analogy, such as filling a gas tank in a car. Discuss the anatomy of eating: how we use our mouths for chewing, our esophagi for swallowing, and our stomachs for digesting. Next, make some small "stomachs" by filling a few stockings with varying degrees of salt. Get out some dolls and strap these stomachs onto the dolls at tummy level. Ask your children questions like, "Which doll's tummy is hungry?" "Which doll is a little full?" and "Which doll is really full?" Then have your children place their hands over their own stomachs and tell you whether they are hungry, a little full, or very full. Finally, go back to the dolls. Ask your children to choose the doll whose stomach matches their own.

Practice this exercise at various times throughout the day so that you catch your kids at different stages of hunger. Do this for a couple of months, as often as your schedule allows. When the researchers did this once a week for four weeks, 70 percent of the children improved their ability to self-regulate, regardless of whether they had started out as undereaters or overeaters.

If making the dolls seems like too much effort (I'm not much of a crafter myself), you can use pictures like the ones shown below to talk to your children about how they feel when they're hungry and full.

This exercise is particularly useful if you are parenting an overeater. When my client Erin introduced her daughter, Kara, to this scale, she found that Kara almost always reported being a 1, even if she had just eaten dinner. That surprised Erin; she had no idea that Kara thought her hunger was so severe. "If you were a one," Erin told Kara, "you would probably feel sick. You wouldn't have enough energy to play or go to school. Is that how you feel?" When Kara

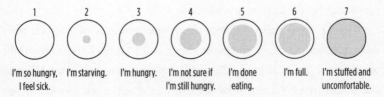

1	2	3	4	5	6	7
I'm so hungry, I feel sick.	I'm starving.	I'm hungry.	I'm not sure if I'm still hungry.	I'm done eating.	I'm full.	I'm stuffed and uncomfortable.

Adapted from *Take the Fight Out of Food* by Donna Fish

said no, Erin followed up with a reassuring statement. "Daddy and I will never let you get that hungry, because we'll always make sure your body has enough food to be healthy." That made Kara think differently about her own hunger. Over time, she started to realize that when she felt hungry she was a 2 or a 3, and that after eating she was almost always a 5. One day I received an email from Erin. She was excited to tell me that Kara was no longer always looking for food. In fact, one night Kara had passed up dessert; she had reported feeling like a 6!

ENCOURAGE THE TRUTH

Here's another radical idea that you might find challenging to accept: You have to let your children eat even when you *know* they aren't hungry. You also have to let your kids stop eating even if you suspect they are not quite full. Otherwise, kids just learn to lie.

Actually, kids aren't really lying; they're just working with the tools we've given them. In most families, if kids want to eat something, they have to say they're hungry, even if they're not. "That cake looks good; I'm hungry." It also means that if they don't want to eat something, kids often have to say they're not hungry, even if they are. "Those peas look gross; I'm not hungry." (This is similar to the way kids also say, "I don't like it," to get out of eating.)

Here's a story that I think will illustrate the problem. One day when my daughter was about four, I needed to drag her along during an unusually long morning of running errands. As we were going to be in a part of town that we rarely visited, which also happened to be near my daughter's favorite ice cream parlor, I told her that I would take her for an ice cream when we were done. After running around for most of the morning, we were headed toward the ice cream parlor. It was around noon, so I asked my daughter if she was hungry. I thought the question was relatively benign, but when my daughter stared back at me in silence, I knew something was wrong.

I waited a moment and then asked again. Still, nothing. After a few minutes I had an insight. "You can't tell me whether you're hungry," I said. "You are worried that if you say you are hungry I will make you eat lunch. Then you'll be too full for ice cream. On the other hand, if you say that you're not hungry, you're worried that I won't let you have any ice cream because we don't usually eat when we're not hungry. Is that right?" My daughter nodded. Her eyes welled up. She was in quite a jam; she really wanted that ice cream.

"How about if you tell me the truth and I promise that you can have ice cream either way?" I offered. That reassured my daughter enough for her to admit, albeit tentatively, that she really was hungry. So I suggested that we stop at a restaurant and share a small salad. After that we would go for the ice cream.

Insisting that kids eat at least some healthy food before moving on to the fun stuff is a common parenting strategy. But I wasn't *using* the ice cream to get my daughter to eat the salad. I was trying to teach her something about hunger. So what would I have done if my daughter had said that she wasn't hungry? If we had the time, I would have pushed off eating for an hour or so until my daughter had more of an appetite. Then we would have eaten the light lunch followed by the ice cream. But if that wasn't in the cards, I would have taken my daughter for the ice cream, as promised. I just would have talked to her about hunger first. "Remember," I would have said, "you're not really hungry. Normally it would be better to wait until you were hungry, but we don't have time today. So let's just have a small ice cream. You don't want to get too full or get a tummy ache."

Eating is a complicated business. If kids are going to be truthful with you about why they want to eat, they need the vocabulary to describe the different reasons people eat. Find a quiet time when your kids are away from food, and talk to them about the different reasons people sometimes choose to eat. Then give your kids some guidance for coping with each of these occasions. For instance, in addition to Tummy Hunger, people often eat because of the following reasons:

- **Taste Hunger:** This can happen when a food looks good. In these circumstances, it's often best to have a small portion, just a taste. Or you can save the food for a time when you're really hungry.

- **Practical Hunger:** You need to eat for practical reasons, such as when there won't be time for lunch later. In this case, you might have to have a few bites even if you aren't hungry.

- **Emotional Hunger:** There are times we want to eat to quench uncomfortable feelings. Teach your kids that it's better to ask for a hug, have a cry, or get some exercise—whatever seems right for the child and the circumstances.

When Melissa had this conversation with her seven-year-old son, Jared, he responded by saying that he felt Taste Hunger all the time, and boy, was he relieved to know that he was normal! Melissa wasn't so relieved. In fact, she was quite upset. When she called me to discuss her next move, I recommended that Melissa stay the course. "Continue helping Jared evaluate why he eats," I said, "and ask him to think about how he feels after he has eaten, especially if he wasn't really hungry." I suggested that Melissa help Jared brainstorm ways to cope with Taste Hunger, being careful not to make him feel guilty (because that would surely encourage him to say he felt Tummy Hunger). Building Jared's awareness would, over time, teach him to cope with his eating.

Becoming more fluent in the language of hunger will stop your kids from gaming the system (by saying they are hungry to get access to food or saying they're not hungry so they can avoid eating). Of course, the only way that can work is if you don't try to talk your kids out of eating if they express the "wrong" kind of hunger. This is particularly important if you are parenting an overeater who worries about food disappearing. But even typical eaters, kids who don't usually worry about their access to food, might resort to saying they're starving if it's the only way you'll let them eat a piece of cake. Over time, kids who learn to lie to their parents also learn to lie to themselves. And that's the real danger here, because lying is just another way that kids get disconnected from what their bodies are telling them about hunger and fullness.

LET EATING ZONES DO THE WORK

Sometimes you can educate your kids about hunger and fullness until you're blue in the face and still have problems getting through dinner. Ivy's three-year-old son, Cole, ate listlessly at dinner. When she checked in with him at the end of the meal—"Are you listening to your tummy?"—he would always say yes and hop down from the table. She would coax him back for some special "Mom time" while she encouraged him to think about his tummy and eat some more. Cole loved the attention, but he rarely ate. Then, thirty minutes later, when he was on his way to bed, Cole would start crying. Like clockwork, Cole was hungry. Ivy usually gave in to her son's last-minute plea for food. Otherwise, she said, the tantrums could go on for hours. What could she do differently?

This is a common problem, and the solution is surprisingly straightforward: Reinforce Eating Zones, and let your structure do the work for you. There were a couple of ways Ivy could use Eating Zones to solve the problem:

- Make dinnertime the final Eating Zone of the day. Ivy could make it clear that there would be no snacks before bed. On the first night, she could explain the rule. If Cole decided not to eat enough dinner and then became hungry, she could say, "This is what I'm talking about. If you don't eat enough food at dinner, you get hungry. I'll give you a snack tonight, but now you know what happens when you don't eat dinner." The next night, she should talk to Cole before dinner again and say, "Remember what happened last night? If you get hungry again tonight, there won't be a snack." And then she would have to stick to her guns. If Cole got hungry, there would be no snack, even if he had a tantrum. Ivy could reassure him that his hunger was temporary and that he'd get something to eat in the morning.

- Create a dinnertime Eating Zone, followed by a snack Eating Zone just before bed. By scheduling a bedtime snack, Ivy would dissolve their power struggle. She wouldn't be so tempted to pressure Cole to eat at dinner. And Cole wouldn't have to throw a tantrum before bed to get something to eat; he'd know the snack was coming. It would be best if Cole's snack were kind of boring—something he liked but didn't love, such as milk or cottage cheese. A treat snack would create incentive to eat less at dinner.

Using the Eating Zones would eliminate the factors that were working against Ivy—pressure, attention, and a control struggle—and produce a better dynamic. Cole needed to know that he couldn't influence when food would and would not be available, even if he had a tantrum. And Ivy needed to know that Cole had plenty of opportunities to eat, *if he wanted to*. Ivy should continue talking to Cole about the link between hunger and eating; eventually he would get it right.

You need to establish strong Eating Zones when you are parenting an overeater, too. One girl, Caroline, always struggled with overeating. No matter how much food was on her plate, she always wanted more. Her mother, Kay, found this extremely frustrating. "I want her to be satisfied with smaller portions," Kay told me. "I know how much a seven-year-old needs to eat, and it's not *that* much." But the more Kay tried to control Caroline's eating—by teaching her about portion size, by limiting the number of servings she could have, by suggesting healthy snacks—the more Caroline seemed to eat. The situation was stressful.

I told Kay she had to turn the question of quantity over to Caroline, but Kay was (understandably) afraid that if she did, Caroline would never stop eating! Then we talked about Eating Zones, and Kay felt a little better. After all, I was not suggesting a free-for-all food fest. "Tell Caroline," I said, "that you are turning over the question of how much she eats to her. Then tell her she can eat as much as she wants, but that she is going to have only three meals and two snacks each day. And let her have some input—show her the Eating Zones schedule and ask if she has suggestions." I stressed that scheduling and food preparation would be the extent of Kay's involvement. Of course, I also encouraged Kay to keep talking to Caroline about the link between hunger and fullness.

One week later, Kay had great news. Caroline hadn't asked for seconds once since the family had implemented this new system. Kay was surprised because the change had happened so quickly. What Kay hadn't realized, though, was that by controlling Caroline's access to food, she had been making Caroline fearful that food would be scarce. As a result, Caroline gorged whenever she had the chance. Providing clear Eating Zones had the opposite effect. Knowing exactly how many times each day she would be able to eat made Caroline feel confident that she was going to have sufficient access to food, and knowing that she could eat as much as she wanted made her giddy.

STRUCTURE: TAKE THE PRESSURE OFF

Eating Zones provide the basic framework for teaching moderation, but there are other structural changes that help you teach your kids how much to eat.

Serve Extremely Small Portions

Serve less food than you expect your kids to eat. Remember the idea of consumption norms: that we eat the amount of food we're used to eating. In our culture, it's better to get kids used to eating less rather than more. Even if you have an undereater, serving less can lead to better eating. One mother I know reversed a pattern of food refusal by giving her daughter the following kinds of meals:

- Three yellow raisins, two oyster crackers, two peas, and three bites of chicken nugget.

- Three small pieces of muffin, three bites of peach, and three bites of hot dog.

These meals may seem ridiculously small, but that's why they worked. Large portions easily overwhelm undereaters, but small portions are liberating. And remember, there are always seconds for kids who are still hungry. Imagine how happy you'll be the first time you hear, "Can I have some more, please?"

Actually, these small meals aren't that far off from the minimum amount that toddlers need to eat. In his book *Touchpoints*, pediatrician T. Berry Brazelton says that the absolute minimum diet for two- and three-year-olds is 1 pint of milk (16 ounces) or the equivalent in cheese, yogurt, or ice cream; 2 ounces of iron-containing protein (meat or an egg) or cereals fortified with iron; 1 ounce of orange juice or fresh fruit; and one multivitamin (to cover for uneaten vegetables).

One way to encourage smaller portions is to let your children dish up their own food. Not only is it fun (young kids seem to love doing this), but it helps children feel more in control. Something else will happen, too. Your kids are more likely to match the serving size to how much they'll eat. When children serve themselves, they are likely to eat about 25 percent less food. No matter whether you have an undereater or an overeater, this is good news, because it means that kids are linking portion sizes to their appetites—not to external "rules" about how much they should eat.

Sometimes, like when you're packing school lunches, you can't provide small portions. Nor can you let your children serve themselves. So what can you do? Consult with your kids! Ask them how much food *they* want to bring to school. Then check in with your children after school to see if you sent the right amount. Make adjustments as necessary and continue checking in with your kids. To ensure there's no pressure, make it clear to your kids that they *never* have to finish all the food you send. And if you're worried your kids have chosen portions that are too small, pack an extra piece of fruit just in case. Tell them, "I'm adding this apple as a backup; you don't have to eat it." If the backup comes back uneaten, you'll know the smaller portion is the right size.

Evaluate Whether Your Child Really Needs a Snack

Kids who snack more eat more. But do they need the additional food? The answer seems to be no. In 2004, a team of researchers studied the eating patterns of a group of four- to six-year-olds, and they discovered that children eat about 40 percent more food and about 30 percent more calories over the course of the day when they eat three snacks compared to days when they skip the snacks entirely. If the children needed the fuel they got from snacks, then they would naturally increase how much they ate at meals on no-snack days; they'd be extra hungry. But they aren't. Kids eat less food and consume fewer calories on no-snack days.

I know that the message that children don't *need* to snack goes against everything you've ever heard, but there's a lot of conflicting evidence out there. And, despite the persistent belief that snacking is a healthy habit, the evidence points in the opposite direction: Today's children typically take in an additional 168 calories from snacks than they did in 1977. (Does this mean that kids are 168 calories hungrier at snack time than they used to be?) Most snack calories come from desserts and sweetened beverages, but salty snacks and candy are the fastest-growing category of snack consumption. When you combine this with the fact that children in other countries, such as France, don't have the same snack habit that American kids do, the practice of snacking becomes even more questionable.

To me, this means that snacking is a philosophy. It's an approach to eating, not a necessity. So feel free to skip the snack if that's what you want to do. If you do decide to let your children snack on a regular basis, make sure you don't let them snack on demand. Not only is it easier to serve healthy snacks when you plan for them, but learning to wait before eating is a key component of learning about moderation.

The Upside of Hunger

Are you comfortable with your children's hunger? Not starvation, but the mild hunger that happens between meals or snacks? A lot of us are Hunger Avoiders, parents who fear *any* hunger. But hunger has an upside:

- Toddlers need to connect the feelings in their tummies with the problem (hunger) and the solution (eating). If they never feel hungry, they never learn this connection.
- When kids start eating when they are *less* hungry, they won't stop until they are *more* full. It's the change in states from start to finish that helps signal satiation.
- Kids who are allowed to get hungry have an easier time distinguishing between physical and emotional hunger because they know what physical hunger feels like.
- Kids who learn they can survive short-term hunger learn that they don't have to fear it. A fear of hunger is what leads many people to overeat.

Don't Rely Too Heavily on Dinner

Rather than fighting with your children to eat more (or differently) at dinner, reduce how important that meal is for your children's health. Consider shifting the heavy-hitter foods (like chicken and vegetables) to lunch or the afternoon snack. Work on making dinnertimes pleasant. Contentious and unpleasant meals make picky eaters even pickier, and that tends to make parents put on the pressure to eat even more.

Allow Some Eating on the Go

You've probably heard that children should always eat at the table, but parenting means managing multiple goals. Sure, you want to teach your children table manners, but you also want them to eat. If you have a child who has trouble eating at the table, consider serving one or two meals a day at the table and everything else to go. Put bite-size bits (which are too small to choke on) on a tray near where your children play (or in a plastic bag they can carry around), and see how much they eat. Sandwiches, fruit, veggies, crackers, and cheese all make great portable foods. As your children mature, you can shift all of their eating to the table.

Help Your Child Eat

Young children are very tired at the end of the day. They may even be too tired to eat. It takes a lot of mental and physical coordination to get the food onto the fork and then to get the fork into the mouth! Consider helping your child by feeding her a few bites, or load up a couple of forkfuls so your child doesn't have to do all the heavy lifting. Check your motivation, though. If you're only trying to get more food into your child, she'll notice and then resist. If your motivation is to be helpful or playful, she'll notice that, too. You might want to help your children eat even if they don't need it; to young children, this is part of the fun of eating together. It's their version of dinnertime conversation.

Practice the Pause

You're pretty sure your child has eaten enough, yet he keeps on going. What can you do? You can tap into the power of the pause.

Pausing. While eating. Gives you a chance. To decide. Whether you want more. Or if grabbing more. Is simply. An automatic. Reflex.

Anything that breaks the eating momentum, even temporarily, can reduce how much we eat. Taking a pause is particularly useful for chronic overeaters, but all children can benefit from learning this style of eating. Start by explaining that it takes some time to feel full from eating and that pausing is a way to let our bodies send our brains the message: "Hey, I'm full; time to quit eating!" Encourage your children to play (or do anything else away from the table) for fifteen or twenty minutes. Finally, check in with your kids after the allotted time. Chances are they'll have forgotten about the food. But if they haven't? Invite them to eat more, even if you think they've had enough.

Downsize the Bites

People tend to eat the same number of food items regardless of their size. When first and sixth graders were offered cookies during an afternoon tea at their school, the children ate fewer grams on the days when the cookies were smaller. In other words, if you're used to eating three cookies, you'll eat three cookies. If those cookies are small cookies, you'll eat less food than if they were large ones.

Rephrase the "Are You Hungry?" Question

When parents want to know whether their children are hungry or full, sometimes they ask only part of the question—either "Are you hungry?" or "Are you full?" These leading questions suggest the answer you hope the child will give.

Instead, ask the whole question: "Are you hungry, or are you full?" This is a balanced, neutral question that lets kids feel free to answer any way they want. It helps them check in with their true physical state and not just say what they think you want to hear.

One–One

Left to their own devices, most children will eat their food in order of diminishing returns: They start with the food they like the best (the pasta), and they end with the food they like the least (the peas). By the time your kids get to the peas, however, they're not terribly hungry anymore, and they are content to stop eating. Either that, or they'll ask for seconds of the stuff they really like. So how do you get your kids to eat their vegetables without undoing your lessons in moderation?

Start by remembering how many fruits and vegetables your kids have already eaten. (Because you implemented the principle of proportion, I bet it's a lot.) Move on to teaching your children this lesson: Because they never know when they'll be full, they need to eat a little of everything the whole time they're eating.

Here's a technique I call One–One. You may remember your mother telling you to eat one bite of everything on your plate, before having a second bite of everything, and so on. Well, that's the technique: one bite of this, one bite of that, going around the plate. (No need to count actual bites; it's the general principle we're after.)

One–One encourages children to eat in a neutral, nonpressuring way. That's the kind of prompt that children are open to hearing. It's also an "equal opportunity strategy," which doesn't make vegetables the "bad guys" and dessert the "good guys." Put a small amount of each food on your child's plate (so the challenge of eating seems doable). Then, during the meal, give your child a gentle reminder, "Remember One–One." What should you do if he refuses? Don't fight about it. Just return to your request the next night. Eventually, One–One will take hold.

In the meantime, if your child asks for seconds of his preferred food without having taken a bite of the food you really want him to eat, don't despair. Give your child seconds. Before you do, though, give this delay tactic a try. "I'll get you seconds in a moment, after I've eaten a little more dinner. In the meantime, why don't you work on those carrots?" Many times children will happily eat a bite or two of vegetable when they know their request for another food is being honored. But even if they don't, remember that moderation lessons are more important than veggie eating.

What Kind of Eating Environment Are You Creating at Home?

Are you inadvertently imitating the obesogenic eating environment of the world around you? Do the sippy cup check. If your children tote around 12-ounce sippy cups that you've filled with apple juice, that cup could deliver more than 150 calories and around 33 grams of sugar. And it teaches your kids to swig big. That's pretty good training for needing that 32-ounce soda later in life!

You can downsize your kids' consumption norms without resorting to drastic measures. According to Cornell researcher Dr. Brian Wansink, here are some things you can do to shape your kids' habits in the direction of moderation:

- Use small plates and cups.
- Instead of eating directly out of a package or box, use small serving bowls and containers, and repackage jumbo boxes into smaller bags.
- At restaurants, split the fries, and order appetizers instead of entrées.

Resist Making the Dessert Deal

Neutralize the power of dessert by letting proportion do the real work. Serve sweets at the end of the meal only occasionally. Then, let everyone eat an appropriate-sized portion, whether or not you think they've earned it.

IF YOU ARE GOOD, YOU CAN HAVE A COOKIE!

Who hasn't resorted to a little behavioral bribe? Food, especially sweets, has the power to produce miraculous results—kids who wait patiently through phone calls, lines at the bank, and even grocery shopping trips that take *forever*. Have you ever heard yourself say, "You can have an ice cream if you play quietly by yourself for another fifteen minutes"?

Resist the urge. When you bribe kids with treats, you send mixed messages about the role that food should play in their lives. So much parental energy goes into encouraging healthy eating, but then we reward our kids for behaving well by giving them . . . brownies!

When parents reward children with dessert, these same children grow into adults who reward themselves with dessert. But it's not just dessert consumption that is affected. People who grow up in families that use food as a reward for success and good behavior are more likely to be excessively concerned about their weight, suffer from weight fluctuations and other problems, such as chronic dieting. A 2003 Yale University study also found that adults who remember their parents using food to control their behavior have higher rates of binge eating. Yikes.

The same goes for using sweets or comfort food to soothe away a child's distress. When your kids get fussy, do you automatically give them something to eat or drink? Do you give your kids something to eat or drink if they're bored or upset, even if you think they're not hungry? This practice comes with a price. Most children lose their appetite when they're upset, but if you routinely use food to solve your children's problems, don't be surprised if your children learn to "fix" their difficult emotions by tucking into a chicken pot pie.

MANAGING SWEETS AND TREATS

The teaching approach assumes that it is generally best to let children decide how much to eat—except when it comes to sweets and treats. In this department, children need some direct guidance. Even Ellyn Satter, the dietician who developed the Division of Responsibility (parents decide *what*; kids decide *how much*), believes that children need a little help learning what an appropriate portion is when it comes to things like dessert, and I agree.

Satter recommends that parents limit kids to eating just one serving of dessert. What's more, she recommends serving dessert at the same time as the main meal to neutralize the power that dessert holds over kids. (For more about Satter's dessert policy, see "Using 'Forbidden' Food" on her website, ellynsatter.com.) I like this strategy, and I take it one step further. Set some guidelines around how often your kids can eat Treat Foods (once a day? three times per week?), and then let your kids decide *when* to indulge. Even if their decision is to eat candy at breakfast.

You may think I'm nuts, but let me explain. For starters, candy isn't any worse for your child in the morning than it is in the afternoon. In fact, a lot of candy has less sugar than some of the items parents regularly dish up in the morning. Two Hersheys Kisses deliver around 5 grams of sugar. In contrast, one serving of Frosted Flakes contains 11 grams, one YoBaby blueberry yogurt has 12 grams, and two Eggo blueberry pancakes have about 7 grams, and that's without the syrup.

But that's not the real reason I advocate letting kids choose to eat some candy in the morning. The benefit of allowing kids to eat candy in the morning—if that is what they want to do—is that it gives kids what they crave most: control. Once your children know how frequently and how much candy they are allowed to consume, and that they get to control when they eat it, the begging and whining will end. If it doesn't, you've got a behavioral problem, not a food problem.

I highly recommend you keep a candy drawer (or a sweets and treats drawer) in your house. It will allow your kids to take ownership of their treat consumption and take the power of treats down a peg or two. The candy drawer is also a great way to cope with party favors (or presents from grandparents, Valentine's Day candy, and so on). Ever notice that your kids want to eat the whole party bag right away, no matter how big it is? When you break up the contents, the candy collection no longer seems like a set. As a result, your kids won't feel entitled to eat it all at once. Then the party bag loses its punch, and your house rules will, well, rule.

I can understand if the idea of a candy drawer makes you panic—"My child will eat all he can stuff into his mouth every chance he gets!"—but remember, you've set the limits. Even if your kids go a little wild with the drawer at first, they will settle down after their access to sweets and treats becomes normal and they develop their self-control.

In the teaching approach, it's less important for parents to strictly monitor how much candy is eaten and more important for kids to learn self-control. In one classic study, a group of four-year-olds were each offered a marshmallow. They were told they could eat the marshmallow right away. However, if they waited ten minutes before eating it, they would be given two marshmallows. Most of the kids chose to eat the single marshmallow, but one-third of the kids waited. Years later, the kids who waited to eat their marshmallows scored an average of 210 points higher on their verbal and math SAT tests than the kids who ate their treats right away! Those scores alone are a reason to help kids develop impulse control. But impulse control also helps kids develop a range of emotional and social skills, such as self-confidence, self-reliance, assertiveness, and being able to cope with adversity and stress.

It's not the candy drawer itself that teaches self-control, so if you really can't stand the idea of having one, feel free to forget about it. You can teach self-control just by involving your kids in the process of choosing when they eat their treats. After you've set the daily or weekly limit, start pointing out upcoming events where there is likely to be junk: "We're going to a party later where there will be cupcakes and candy. You can have a doughnut now, but then you can't have the treats later. Which do you want?"

One woman I know had a struggle with her kids almost every Thursday. In their family, Thursday was doughnut-for-breakfast day. When she picked her children up after school they often asked for an additional treat. If Mom said no, the kids complained until she gave in. After Mom started explaining that the kids could choose between the doughnuts and the cookies, they happily lived with their decisions.

Even young children can participate in making their treat choices. Of course, young children are more likely to choose now instead of later, but that is not a reason to delay including kids in the decision-making process. You will actually help them develop their self-control. Young children are also more likely to forget in the afternoon that they've already had their treat in the morning. So don't expect your kids to remember their choice. Give your kids some kind of visual cue—like a chart or a refrigerator magnet—to remind them of how many candies they're allowed and how many they've consumed.

Finally, if you want to break the allure that Treat Foods have over kids, try this suggestion from Ellyn Satter: On occasion, offer your children unlimited access to sweets and treats. The free-for-all isn't actually unlimited; it's confined to the amount a child can consume in one sit-down snacking session. When forced to sit at the table, most young children run out of attention before they run out of steam. Stomach space is limited, but attention span is even more so. It's a brilliant, self-limiting system! And when kids are sometimes allowed this kind of indulgence, they aren't as preoccupied with mooching treats the rest of the time.

CELEBRATIONS

There are plenty of times when your child will be exposed to an overflowing banquet of food options. Thanksgiving and Halloween come to mind; so do church socials or even visits to Grandma's house. Parents with a nutrition mindset try to get kids to eat the healthy stuff before they go for the Fun Foods or the Treat Foods. This makes parents feel better, but it teaches kids to overeat.

Let's be honest. At Thanksgiving dinner, nobody passes up the pie, even kids who have filled up on healthy foods. (Unless they don't really like pie, in which case they go for the other treats.) You end up with kids who don't just celebrate; they gorge themselves. So what can you do? Think of holidays as big buffets.

Buffets are challenging eating environments, where many people overindulge. So many choices, so much food! Remember Brian Wansink, the researcher from Cornell University whose ideas for downsizing consumption norms I listed earlier in the chapter? A few years ago he and a colleague studied how people approach buffets. They discovered that some people browse buffets before serving themselves; others begin loading up at once and don't stop until they reach the end. The browsers tended to be thinner than the loaders. The researchers never asked the eaters why they chose one serving method over the other, but I think it's safe to say that the browsers scanned the buffet as a way to make sure they filled their plates with their favorite foods before their plates were filled to capacity or beyond.

Use big food events to teach your kids how to be browsers, not loaders. Tell them that during parties and on food-focused holidays, we worry a little less about proportion. On these occasions, it's OK to enjoy the special foods, as long you don't eat too much. Tiny tummies fill up fast, so when your tykes start wolfing down the pretzels and pizza at birthday parties, help them learn to pace themselves by reminding them of all the food to come. On the other hand, if you've got kids who would prefer to go straight to cake, let them. It's not as if pizza is healthy—and even if it were, telling kids that healthy food is the barrier to fun teaches them the wrong lesson.

You can even teach a browsing strategy for Halloween. Let your children browse their haul and eat what they like, but remind them to pay attention to their tummies. (I often say that the only rule is "Don't throw up.") Then dump the rest into the candy drawer. This is the only way to solve the Halloween problem. If you take away the candy or severely restrict its access, your children won't learn a thing about how to handle this holiday eating mess, and you'll be left fighting over candy year after year.

Because holidays and parties are a nonnegotiable part of child-hood, you might as well use them to teach your kids the habit of moderation. After all, wouldn't you be happier—and maybe even a little bit healthier—if you had learned the right party habits when you were a kid? So set your kids up for a lifetime of healthy eating by teaching them how to party while they're young. Then sit back and let the good times roll.

Troubleshooting

From raising my child and after talking to hundreds of other parents, I have learned that just when you think you've got your new feeding structure in place, something pops up to challenge it. You're psyched about teaching your child to taste new foods, but when you offer her a teeny sample of minced olive, she shrieks like a banshee on fire. You explain to your son that there will be some limits around sweets and treats, and he goes along with the plan for a while, but then he suddenly begins whining for candy the moment he wakes up. Your kids get sick. You get tired. You cook up some reliable old favorites, and no one in your family will eat any of them.

Believe me, the teaching approach works. But it doesn't work all at once, and it doesn't necessarily come naturally to those of us who have been trapped inside the nutrition mindset for years. That's why I've presented the teaching approach so that each step builds on the previous one. You can learn the separate concepts and incorporate them into your family's lifestyle as slowly as you like and in a way that works for you. These steps might not feel normal at first. Switching from the nutrition mindset to a teaching approach can sometimes be tough going. The nutrition approach is such an engrained—ahem—*habit* that you may find yourself periodically reverting to old ways. Your kids and spouse may long for the old system, too. Habits are so hard to change! So expect some ups, some downs, and some shockers. They happen to everyone.

It helps to remember that teaching kids to eat right is a process, not something you do once and then you're done. You might think of this as the bad news. The good news is that it definitely gets easier as both you and your children become more accustomed to the new structure, as you learn new parenting skills, and as your children learn new eating skills. Still, to stay on top of the process you'll need to constantly tweak the system, revise your message, and keep talking to your children. It'll help, too, if you think of every problem as a teaching opportunity and not something that just ruined the good thing you (finally) had going or as evidence that nothing you do will ever really change how your kids eat. Teaching children to eat right is like slowly peeling an onion; you feel as if you are going around in circles, but every time you visit a familiar spot you're actually one step closer to the core, or in this case, to your goal.

As you work toward that goal, take some time along the way to acknowledge your accomplishments. Of course, you ultimately want your children to learn a style of eating that emphasizes the three habits of proportion, variety, and moderation. But your kids don't need to have these habits down pat before you can start celebrating. In fact, it's best if you recognize and rejoice in each small step. It will encourage both you and your kids to carry on.

And your children's eating habits aren't the only places to look for signs of progress. You can find evidence of growth by looking at *all* the lessons your kids have been learning. Remember, sometimes these lessons take a long time to translate into eating habits. One little girl I know, a child who has a tendency to overeat, has a mountain of lessons to learn before she'll truly know how to eat right. She has to figure out how to manage what seems to her like an insatiable appetite, a burgeoning weight and health crisis, feelings of shame and remorse, and a family culture that sends her mixed messages. She also needs to tap into her internal hunger and satiation cues, to differentiate *those* feelings from other emotional feelings, and to figure out how to navigate a world filled with tempting treats. As if that weren't enough, in order for any of this to happen, her parents need to learn a new style of parenting, too. Should this family wait for the end result to feel good about their hard work? Absolutely not! And neither should you. Celebrate every step of the way. You and your kids have earned it.

When you do experience bumps in the road, don't give up. Regroup. Step back. Reexamine the structure you have in place. Take a fresh look at the lessons your children need to learn, and ask yourself if you are teaching the lessons that you're intending to teach. The rest of this chapter diagnoses some common problems parents run into and pinpoints solutions. Often you'll find that a simple fix is all you need to get things back on track.

DIAGNOSIS: YOU'RE ASKING YOUR CHILD TO TAKE A STEP THAT'S TOO BIG

One of the primary reasons parents fail to see the results they desire is that they present their children with a challenge that is simply too big. If you find yourself struggling to make progress, ask yourself if there is any way you can break the task you're trying to teach your child into smaller increments. Let's say you want your child to start eating more vegetables (and to do it without always having to be nudged). Before he can do that, he'll have to learn the principle of proportion and learn to eat a wider variety of flavors and textures. Before he can do that, he'll have to learn to taste new foods. And before he can learn *that*, he'll have to trust that he'll never be forced to eat anything he doesn't want to eat. Remember, baby steps are always easier to master than giant steps, and mastery builds confidence, which leads to more success.

DIAGNOSIS: YOUR STRUCTURE IS INCONSISTENT

Another reason many parents struggle is that they implement their new feeding structure inconsistently. They start using the Rotation Rule, for instance, and then, after an initial burst of enthusiasm, they begin to slack off. Why does this happen? Because change is hard. Most systems—family systems included—seek to maintain a state of constancy (or homeostasis). The familiar pattern of interactions that families develop creates a sense of order and normalcy, both for parents and for kids. And, just like a mobile hanging over a baby's crib that automatically starts to right itself when you pull on one side of it, members of a family often seek to right the system when someone introduces change. This is one way to understand the pushback you might have gotten from your kids when you implemented any of the techniques offered in this book; your children are trying to reestablish their sense of order. A desire for homeostasis also explains why parents often implement strategies inconsistently; they want to reestablish *their* sense of order (the old problems may have been disturbing, but at least they were familiar).

The trouble with implementing change inconsistently, besides the fact that every time you do things the *old* way you're not doing things the *new* way, is that the inconsistency teaches your kids the wrong sorts of lessons. (It always comes back to the lessons!) Every time you interact with your children around food, you're not only teaching them what, when, why, and how much to eat but also teaching them how to relate to you.

When parents are inconsistent, their children learn these lessons:

- Rules don't need to be taken seriously.

- Parents can't be trusted to do what they say.

- Rebelling is a successful strategy that sometimes (or even usually) gets kids what they want.

In this way, inconsistency intensifies whatever problem parents are attempting to resolve. And every go-round solidifies *these* lessons, making eating problems seem even more intractable.

The solution to inconsistency is obvious: Become more consistent. Sometimes this is relatively easy to do. In many cases, all that is required is just a little more advance work. Maybe, to implement proportion more consistently, you need a better stash of healthy snacks. And maybe you even need to keep these snacks in the car. (After all, fruit doesn't need to be refrigerated.) Or maybe you need to rehearse how you are going to respond to your child's pushback so you don't instinctually revert to your old ways. When my client Kristen found herself giving in to her son Zach's demands for snacks, a practice she knew was undermining her efforts to implement Eating Zones, we developed a set of stock statements that she could use to keep herself on track.

To herself, Kristen could say any or all of the following: "Zach couldn't have been that hungry if he skipped dinner." "He'll have a bedtime snack in twenty minutes; that's not really very long. He's going to be OK." "By helping Zach learn that he can live with temporary hunger, I'm teaching him a valuable life lesson about food and eating." "Reinforcing this boundary is good authoritative parenting." "The more consistent I am, the more quickly Zach will accept the new structure."

To Zach she could say, "I know you're not happy waiting until snack time because you're hungry right now, but feeling hungry is what happens when you skip dinner," or "We'll have a snack in twenty minutes but not while you're having a tantrum," or "I know you're really angry because I'm making you wait before having a snack. But it's not OK to scream or throw things when you're mad. You can use words to tell me how you feel."

If you find yourself caught off guard by your child's reactions, practice what you'll say and do to reinforce your rules. And here's a hint: The reactions that you find the most difficult are going to be the ones that bump up against your issues the most. That's why they're so problematic. Try rereading Chapter 3 to identify your emotional trigger points. It will also help you brainstorm solutions you can use to shore up your feeding structure.

Sometimes, though, parents have a hard time being consistent because they're trying to change too many things at once. That's why I often advise scaling back on your ambitions, not your long-term hopes and dreams (keep those firmly intact). Rather, I suggest viewing inconsistency as a sign that you've tried to tackle too much change in too short of a time. To understand why, let's go back to thinking about that mobile hanging over a baby's crib.

Imagine that mobile: It has four arms, and dangling from each arm is a cute little monkey. Each monkey is a different size and is hanging from a different length of wire. Still, the monkeys are perfectly balanced to maintain the mobile's equilibrium. Let's say you've decided to replace one of the monkeys with a different animal, perhaps a lamb. To do that you would have to calibrate (and then possibly recalibrate) how big or heavy the lamb needs to be, and how long or short the hanging wire needs to be, to keep the mobile from becoming lopsided. It might not take that long or require that much effort. But even if it did, because you were working on replacing only one monkey, you could focus all of your attention on what you were doing. You could anticipate how the lamb would throw the mobile off balance, and you could make adjustments accordingly. Moreover, because you were working on only one arm of the mobile, it's highly unlikely that even if the mobile became unbalanced it would go crashing to the floor.

But what would happen if you tried to replace two of the monkeys, or even three of them? Or if you were working with a multitiered mobile? Your ability to anticipate, and then repair, the effect of each replacement on the mobile as a whole would be hampered by the sheer volume of the task. And the chances that you could balance the mobile before it started to get completely tangled, and possibly even fall apart, would become increasingly smaller with each change you introduced. You might tinker with the mobile for a while, but it probably wouldn't take long before you decided to give up. "Mobiles," you might think, "are not all they're cracked up to be!"

The "mobile" my client Yasmin has been trying to balance for the past few years is very complicated. Yasmin's son, Shawn, is a strong-willed child who seems to delight in challenging Yasmin on every front. Shawn never wants to eat the food that is served, he doesn't want to come to the table, and he constantly demands cookies for snack. Sometimes he'll try new foods, but most often Shawn clamps his mouth shut and refuses to budge from his position of refusal. What's more, Shawn is one of those slight children who doesn't seem to care if he ever eats. That gives him a distinct advantage over Yasmin, who cares a great deal about how much Shawn eats.

Every three or four months, Yasmin calls me to say that she's ready to gear up to improve Shawn's eating habits—once again. Although we always focus our conversations on one behavior that Shawn needs to learn, Yasmin wants *everything* to change. She's too impatient to take things slowly. So Yasmin sets about implementing Eating Zones *and* the Rotation Rule, she enforces good behavior at the table, and she stops caving in to Shawn's demands for cookies (serving a fruit snack instead). For a time, Yasmin keeps the

Improving Parenting Skills Can Improve Children's Health

People who practice authoritative parenting are more likely to have children who are healthy eaters; this you know. Until now, though, most researchers had assumed this relationship existed because authoritative parents are more likely to set limits around *food* and to respond to their children's food-related desires with warmth and compassion. Now, however, a study published in the journal *Pediatrics* shows that children eat better when their parents improve their parenting skills *in general*. In this study, youths whose parents participated in a series of skill-building workshops when the kids were four years old had lower body mass index (BMI) scores and improved health behaviors (better eating habits, more physical activity, less sedentary screen time) as they approached adolescence. These skill-building workshops didn't even address nutrition, activity, or weight; they were designed to reduce behavioral problems. What the researchers discovered, though, is that teaching parents to be responsive and nurturing, to set limits, to enforce discipline, and to promote positive behavior is a strategy that pays off in many different ways. Including eating.

system balanced: She corrects and encourages Shawn on all fronts, and his behavior slowly begins to improve. But then, Yasmin makes one exception to the Rotation Rule (she's tired and Shawn wants pizza again), and then another. She starts to ignore the Eating Zones (Shawn wants cookies, and she wants some peace and quiet). And before Yasmin knows what is happening, Shawn is back to his old contrary self, and the system has been derailed.

I'm not blaming Yasmin. I applaud her resolve to keep working on these problems, especially in the face of what feels to her like constant defeat. But I'm also not surprised by her struggles. She's taken on too much change at once. If this sounds like what's happened to you, just scale back. Reassess your situation and pick only one issue to work on. This will help focus your limited time and energy. It'll help your kids, too. They won't feel as though their entire world has turned upside down. And, just like a hanging mobile that won't swing frantically in response to a tender tap, your kids will respond more gently to change that feels more moderate.

DIAGNOSIS: YOU AREN'T TALKING TO YOUR KIDS

Have you been talking to your kids? Many parents overlook this step. Or if they do talk to their children, they focus most of the conversation on the food. "Apples are good for you." "Those chips have too many calories." To be successful, though, you have to talk to your kids about the new eating structure. You also have to talk about the reasons behind the changes. Then you have to solicit input from your kids so that you know how they feel about the changes and so they feel like they're part of the team. Of course, you also have to be clear about what types of behavior are acceptable and what behaviors will result in some consequences.

Think your kids are too young for this kind of conversation? They're not. Experts say that most kids start to grasp the concept of consequences for their actions somewhere between eighteen months and two years of age. But I say, even if your children don't fully understand the connection between actions and consequences, you should still talk to them about this link. It's how they'll learn.

There isn't anything you need your children to understand about eating right that can't be presented in child-size nuggets. For instance, Mary wrote to me because she was having a problem that many parents can relate to. Her two-year-old son, Bobby, goes to a daycare center where the kids are fed macaroni and cheese, corn dogs, and even Pop-Tarts. Every day, when Bobby comes home, he says he is starving. And every day he starts whining for cookies, crackers, and candy. "What's happened to my child?" Mary began to wonder, "the one who loved fruits and vegetables?" Now, every time Mary offers Bobby an apple after school, he throws a fit and refuses to eat it.

How can she turn things around? The answer: Start talking to Bobby.

Some lessons can't be learned by structure alone. They need explanation. Imagine walking into your child's classroom to find the teacher handing each child a book. Afterward, you watch the teacher sit down in her chair, open her book, and start reading quietly to herself. It wouldn't take long before the children figured out what they were supposed to do: Open their books and start reading. So far the teacher's actions seem perfectly adequate; the children have all the information they need to figure out what they're supposed to do. Now imagine that the children don't know how to read. Do you still think the teacher's actions seem adequate? Probably not. Some lessons need active instruction.

To learn to eat (and to behave) differently when he gets home from daycare, Bobby needs more than an apple. He needs to learn about the concept of proportion, and he needs to learn the consequences of his decisions. The conversation Mary might have with Bobby could go something like this:

MARY: *The food you eat at daycare is pretty tasty, isn't it?*

BOBBY: *Yeah, I love it.*

MARY: *I love that kind of food, too. But you know what? It's not the healthiest food.*

BOBBY: *It's not?*

MARY: *No. Remember how I always say that we have to eat things like fruits and vegetables more often than we eat hot dogs, noodles, and cookies?*

BOBBY: *Yeah.*

MARY: *Well, because you eat all that Fun Food and Treat Food during the day, we have to be extra careful to eat Growing Food at home. That's why I am always going to offer you things like apples and pears for a snack when you get home from school. You don't have to eat the snack, but there won't be food again until dinner. OK?*

BOBBY: *OK, but I don't like pears. They're mushy.*

MARY: *I didn't know you don't like pears. Thanks for telling me. This must be new because you liked pears last week. Let's make up a list of the fruit you like right now, and I'll make sure to include those items in our Rotation Rule. OK?*

BOBBY: *OK.*

MARY: *But remember, I'm going to keep serving pears from time to time. I like them, and you never know when you might want to start eating them again.*

If you're worried that having this kind of conversation with a young child would make him feel bad about his daycare center, as if you're somehow putting it down or accusing staff of serving unhealthy food, you could add something like, "Every family eats differently, and your teachers have to make sure they serve something that everyone likes," or "Your teachers know that kids like to eat Fun Foods and Treat Foods with their friends. But we can't eat those foods all the time."

The key to authoritative parenting is blending a solid structure and firm discipline with warmth and compassion. That's why

Has a Strategy Backfired?

Sometimes techniques, even ones that are well designed, end up teaching a lesson that's the opposite of the one you intend. That's because there's no one-size-fits-all strategy when it comes to kids. You've always got to look at the feeding system through *your* child's eyes. For instance, I've suggested that a good way to increase how many vegetables your kids eat is to serve veggies first, when there are no other competing foods on the table. When my client Samantha tried this technique, however, it didn't work. We examined the situation from her daughter's perspective and saw that by staging meals in courses (so that vegetables weren't competing with preferred foods), Alice wasn't learning to eat her veggies. Instead, she was learning that the good stuff always came last! If she just waited long enough, Alice knew she could eat the food she *really* liked. To get the result Samantha desired, she had to change tactics. In this instance, I recommended that Samantha serve small portions of everything at once and then teach Alice the technique I call One–One (discussed on page 215). With this approach, Alice learned the right lesson, and her veggie intake began to increase.

talking to your children is so crucial. It's where the warmth and compassion come in. During these conversations, not only do you get to explain your thinking to your children but your kids get to explain *their* thinking to *you*. It's during these conversations that you can actively incorporate some of their goals and objectives into the plan, and also hash out the time for appropriate choices.

DIAGNOSIS: YOU'VE BROKEN TRUST WITH YOUR KIDS

It can be painful for parents to recognize the extent to which they've broken trust with their children. Often, though, this is the crux of whatever feeding problem they're having. When children are tricked into eating foods they don't want to eat, when they are told to eat a few more bites only to find out they have to eat even a few more bites, or when they are made to feel guilty for eating less than (or more than, or differently from) what their parents feel is right, they learn to feel wary—both about food and about their parents in relation to food. If you (and your children) experience tension around eating, there's a good chance that you need to rebuild trust. The more tension there is in your household, and the longer that tension has existed, the more you need to talk. A lot is being said in the silence.

I know the impact of breaking trust (even just a little), and the importance of reestablishing it, from firsthand experience. When my daughter was about four years old, I made her swallow a bite of mushroom. I don't know why. All I can say is that she'd been eating mushrooms for years. (One time she ate the entire batch of mushrooms I was sautéing to put into a quiche. We ate a broccoli quiche that night!) On this one day, however, my daughter said she didn't like mushrooms. Instead of lightly accepting this new food preference—by letting her go on strike, for instance—I said something more like, "What? You like mushrooms. You always eat mushrooms. I made this dish the way you like it. *Now eat it.*" She looked up at me with what I now think were pitiful eyes (but which at the time I thought were defiant eyes) and started to swallow. Only she didn't swallow. She gagged. I, of course, saw that as more defiance and tried again: "Swallow it." She responded with more gagging.

I can't say that was my finest parenting moment. I can say, though, that it was one of my biggest learning moments. For days after the mushroom incident, my daughter was a wary eater. She approached new foods tentatively, and during mealtimes, she looked at me with frightened eyes. She no longer trusted that *she* was in charge of what she ate or that the dinner table was a safe place.

And then we talked. I apologized for what I'd done and promised never to make her eat anything ever again. And I haven't! During the conversation we also talked about her feelings, about the food, about the fear she felt toward me, and about the gagging. Slowly, over the next few days, my happy, adventurous eater returned to the table. (Though her mushroom-eating days, sadly, seem to be over.)

Lack of trust is a bigger problem than many parents realize. Think about how much courage it takes for children to change how they eat. That is why I always recommend that parents precede any changes to their feeding routine with an honest conversation like the one I had with my daughter, one that doesn't just include where they've been and where they're going, but that builds their family bonds as well.

ARE YOU OVERWHELMED BY TEACHING HABITS TO MULTIPLE CHILDREN?

Sometimes people get nuts thinking about how to incorporate the structure of The Big Fix into a family with multiple kids. How, they wonder, can they implement the Rotation Rule *and* give choices without becoming a full-time personal chef? The answer is to make a few executive decisions that the whole family has to live with (this is what we're eating tonight), to give choices when possible (would you like cereal or eggs for breakfast? I'm happy to prepare either), and then to rotate through choices so that each person sometimes gets what he wants (I fixed Timmy's favorite meal today; tomorrow I'll fix yours). One woman I know gives each member of her family (parents included) one "restaurant ticket" that enables that person to choose which restaurant the family goes to on the nights the parents decide the group will eat out. Tickets are turned in after they are used, and when every family member has used his or her ticket, they are redistributed.

Parents often worry that one child's food preferences or picky eating will spread like a virus to the other children. You can prevent this contagion from occurring by identifying the specific lessons that siblings need to learn. Here are a few:

- **Sometimes your brother gets to eat his favorite food and you don't.** (This is a variation on the "You can't eat your favorite food every single night" rule that all children need to learn.)

- *Fair* **doesn't mean that everyone gets to eat the same thing at the same time, especially when it comes to sweets and treats.** *Fair* **means people get treats when the time is right for them.**

In other words, instead of teaching that *everyone* gets cookies
if *anyone* gets cookies, teach your kids that if they've already
eaten their cookies (at school for instance) but their brother
hasn't, he can have a cookie for dessert, but they can't.

- **You don't have to like what I serve, but you do have to be
  polite.** Parents are inclined to give their picky eaters a pass
  on what they say about food. This can be a mistake, especially if other children follow the complainer's lead. It's fine
  (actually, it's great) to encourage your children to express
  their opinions about what you serve, especially if you encourage them to use any of the "Two Hundred (or so) Tantalizing
  Words" from Chapter 6, but outbursts, tantrums, or other
  disruptive behavior is out of line. You can explain this concept pretty easily: "I'm sure you didn't mean to hurt my feelings, but I worked hard on cooking this. If you don't want

"My Child Would Rather Entertain Than Eat"

Everyone loves the class clown. Clowns make things fun; they
entertain; they make us happy. Unless, that is, you're trying to
get something done. Like teach a class or serve some dinner. If
you've got a clown on your hands, implement this ten-point
plan for feeding an entertainer. (Notice the plan uses a blend of
Eating Zones, strategies for implementing proportion, and
some new techniques developed just for this situation.)

1. Talk to your child about the importance of eating at mealtimes, and acknowledge that eating rather than entertain-
   ing can be difficult and boring. Brainstorm solutions *with*
   your child, including some of the following suggestions.

2. Give your child ten minutes of premeal or postmeal attention every night, so he can revel in having an audience.

3. Limit snacks before dinner so your child is hungry when he sits down to dine. Alternatively, consider giving your child a quality premeal snack (fruit, vegetables, salad, etc.) so you know he's good to go, even if he never really settles down to dinner.

4. Teach your child to share the stage by giving everyone time to talk during meals. Consider using a talking stick to promote table-time democracy with a visual cue of who has the floor.

5. Set some of the conversation by introducing a topic for discussion: politics, world affairs, geography, or the pros and cons of something that's on your mind.

6. Require everyone to stay seated for the duration of the meal (even if standing would really, really enhance the story).

7. Decide, with your child, how much time he should have to complete his meal *after* the last other person has finished eating. Five or ten minutes is appropriate. Use a timer if you think it will help.

8. Give your child gentle reminders throughout the meal to let him know how much eating time he has left.

9. Eliminate after-dinner snacks.

10. Remember to enjoy the nightly show!

to eat it you don't have to, but let's be polite. And remember, other people at the table are enjoying their food. Let's not make them feel bad about eating it."

- **Difference rocks.** This isn't a food-focused lesson; it's a life lesson. We look different. We have different ideas. We wear different clothes, enjoy different sports, and yes, enjoy eating different foods. Point out food preferences that no one can feel bad about. "I like chocolate ice cream. You like vanilla." Empowering difference is a way of empowering kids.

- **Preferences can change.** Knowing that children's taste preferences go through stages isn't something just for parents to know; kids can benefit from knowing this, too. The more you matter-of-factly state this truth, the less your children will be influenced to refuse food like their siblings do. "John just hasn't tasted the rice enough times yet," is a great way to frame one person's food preferences for young children. "I didn't like rice when I was young. Now I love it. That's why it's important to keep tasting."

THE TEACHING APPROACH: A SOLUTION FOR EVERY PROBLEM

The thing I love most about the teaching approach is that it empowers parents to transform *any* feeding challenge into a step toward good eating habits. Unlike the nutrition mindset, which gives parents a one-size-fits-all set of static recommendations about food (with menus to memorize and portions to measure), the teaching approach is a dynamic strategy that can be used with different children, at different times, and in different situations. It doesn't matter whether your kids present you with a small hitch or a complete curve ball. The teaching approach will help you determine the appropriate solution. In other words, you now have a realistic plan for living in the real world.

Many parents blanch at the idea of having to be mindful about the lessons underlying *every* feeding interaction. I understand; it can seem like an overwhelming task, one that requires too much attention. But these same parents find that the teaching approach, like exercising, gets easier the more they do it. Not just because this "muscle" gets stronger but because, with practice, more of their feeding interactions teach the *right* lessons. Over time, then, there are fewer and fewer lessons—and therefore fewer and fewer feeding problems—to correct.

The strategies in this book may be simple, but they're not necessarily easy. They take work and commitment on your part, not to mention on the part of your kids as they practice new skills. But the benefits are great. Children who can successfully manage their own eating are at a huge advantage as they negotiate the food world. And don't forget the fact that you'll no longer spend time trying to get your kids to eat more or to eat better. They'll be doing it with you. That's why it's not about the broccoli; it's about habits. By providing an environment in which your children feel empowered and knowledgeable (not controlled or pressured), you're setting them up for a lifetime of healthy and happy eating. And that was your goal all along!

NOTES

All product information was obtained from manufacturers' websites and was accurate at the time of writing.

CHAPTER 1

On any given day: Fox, M. K., E. Condon, R. R. Briefel, K. Reidy, and D. M. Deming. "Food Consumption Patterns of Young Preschoolers: Are They Starting Off on the Right Path?" *Journal of the American Dietetic Association* 110, no. 12, suppl. 3 (2010): S52–S59.

Yet almost every preschooler; On average, children reach: Piernas, C., and B. M. Popkin. "Trends in Snacking Among U.S. Children." *Health Affairs* 29, no. 3 (2010): 398–404.

When children do eat vegetables; Compared to preschoolers: Lorson, B. A., H. R. Melgar-Quinonez, and C. A. Taylor. "Correlates of Fruit and Vegetable Intakes in US Children." *Journal of the American Dietetic Association* 109, no. 3 (2009): 474–478.

Nearly 40 percent: Reedy, J., and S. M. Krebs-Smith. "Dietary Sources of Energy, Solid Fats, and Added Sugars Among Children and Adolescents in the United States." *Journal of the American Dietetic Association* 110, no. 10 (2010): 1477–1484.

Some researchers worry: Parker-Pope, T. "U.S. Children: Generation Snack." *Well* (blog). *New York Times*, March 2, 2010. well.blogs.nytimes.com/2010 /03/02/u-s-children-generation-snack.

The Centers for Disease Control and Prevention reports: Centers for Disease Control and Prevention. "Data and Statistics." In *Overweight and Obesity.* Last updated January 11, 2013. cdc.gov/obesity/data/childhood.html.

About 25 percent of overweight: Centers for Disease Control and Prevention. "Tips for Parents: Ideas to Help Children Maintain a Healthy Weight." In *Healthy Weight—It's Not a Diet, It's a Lifestyle!* Last updated October 31, 2011. cdc.gov/healthyweight/children.

Children today have a thirty: Centers for Disease Control and Prevention, U.S. Department of Health & Human Services. "Nutrition and the Health of Young People." 2008. cdc.gov/HealthyYouth/nutrition/pdf/facts.pdf.

Scientists predict that today's children: Olshansky, S. J., D. J. Passaro, R. C. Hershow, et al. "A Potential Decline in Life Expectancy in the United States in the 21st Century." *New England Journal of Medicine* 352, no. 11 (2005): 1138–1145.

Moreover, the nutrition mindset teaches: Raghunathan, R., R. Walker Naylor, and W. D. Hoyer. "The Unhealthy = Tasty Intuition and Its Effects on Taste Inferences, Enjoyment, and Choice of Food Products." *Journal of Marketing* 70 (2006): 170–184.

Healthy food tastes bad: Werle, C. O. C., O. Trendel, and G. Ardito. "*Unhealthy* Food Is Not Tastier for Everybody: The '*Healthy=Tasty*' French Intuition." *Food Quality and Preference* 28 (2013): 116–121.

Recently, a collaborative team of French: Saulais, L., M. Doyon, B. Ruffieux, and H. Kaiser. "Consumer Knowledge About Dietary Fats: Another French Paradox?" *British Food Journal* 114, no. 1 (2012): 108–120.

The book: Ernsperger, L., and T. Stegen-Hanson. *Just Take a Bite: Easy, Effective Answers to Food Aversions and Eating Challenges!* Arlington, TX: Future Horizons, 2004.

Yet the USDA notes in its document: U.S. Department of Agriculture. "MyPyramid Food Guidance System Education Framework." 2005. choosemyplate.gov/food-groups/downloads/MyPyramid_education _framework.pdf.

CHAPTER 2

Sufficient calcium: Office of Dietary Supplements. National Institutes of Health. "Dietary Supplement Fact Sheet: Calcium." Reviewed March 14, 2013. ods. od.nih.gov/factsheets/Calcium-HealthProfessional.

Some research suggests that sugar: Burger, K. S., and E. Stice. "Frequent Ice Cream Consumption Is Associated with Reduced Striatal Response to Receipt of an Ice Cream-Based Milkshake." *American Journal of Clinical Nutrition* 95, no. 4 (2012): 810–817.

Did you know that drinking: Ludwig, D. S., K. E. Peterson, and S. L. Gortmaker. "Relation between Consumption of Sugar-Sweetened Drinks and Childhood Obesity: A Prospective, Observational Analysis." *Lancet* 357 (2001): 505–508.

the problem of cream cheese: Center for Nutrition Policy and Promotion. U.S. Department of Agriculture. "Got Your Dairy Today? 10 Tips to Help You Eat and Drink More Fat-Free or Low-Fat Dairy Foods." DG TipSheet No. 5. June 2011. choosemyplate.gov/food-groups/downloads/TenTips/DGTip sheet5GotYourDairyToday.pdf.

Children now consume more than; On average, children consume: Piernas, C., and B. M. Popkin. "Trends in Snacking among U.S. Children." *Health Affairs* 29, no. 3 (2010): 398–404.

Manufacturers have found: Kessler, D. A. *The End of Overeating: Taking Control of the Insatiable American Appetite.* New York: Rodale, 2009.

It's easy to see why one team: Orrell-Valente, J. K., L. G. Hill, W. A. Brechwald, et al. "'Just Three More Bites': An Observational Analysis of Parents' Socialization of Children's Eating at Mealtime." *Appetite* 48, no. 1 (2007): 37–45.

One study of college students: Batsell, W. R. Jr., A. S. Brown, M. E. Ansfield, and G. Y. Paschall. "'You Will Eat All of That!': A Retrospective Analysis of Forced Consumption Episodes." *Appetite* 38 (2002): 211–219.

Instead of looking inward: Hodges, E. A., S. O. Hughes, J. Hopkinson, and J. O. Fisher. "Maternal Decisions About the Initiation and Termination of Infant Feeding." *Appetite* 50 (2008): 333–339.

More than one-third: Centers for Disease Control and Prevention. "Childhood Obesity Facts." In *Adolescent and School Health.* Last updated July 10, 2013. cdc.gov/healthyyouth/obesity/facts.htm.

In her book: Nestle, M. *What to Eat.* New York: North Point Press, 2006.

CHAPTER 3

Researchers who study brain: Siegel, D. J., and T. P. Bryson. *The Whole-Brain Child: 12 Revolutionary Strategies to Nurture Your Child's Developing Mind.* New York: Bantam Books, 2011.

In Jennifer's defense: Flood-Obbagy, J. E., and B. J. Rolls. "The Effect of Fruit in Different Forms on Energy Intake and Satiety at a Meal." *Appetite* 52 (2009): 416–422.

You might be teaching your children: Stifter, C. A., S. Anzman-Frasca, L. L. Birch, and K. Voegtline. "Parent Use of Food to Soothe Infant/Toddler Distress and Child Weight Status. An Exploratory Study." *Appetite* 57 (2011): 693–699.

It's that they also end up confusing: Blissett, J., E. Haycraft, and C. Farrow. "Inducing Preschool Children's Emotional Eating: Relations with Parental Feeding Practices." *American Journal of Clinical Nutrition* 92 (2010): 359–365.

CHAPTER 4

Pushy or controlling parents: Blissett, J. "Relationships Between Parenting Style, Feeding Style and Feeding Practices and Fruit and Vegetable Consumption in Early Childhood." *Appetite* 57 (2011): 826–831.

When a team of Pennsylvania: Carper, J. L., J. O. Fisher, and L. L. Birch. "Young Girls' Emerging Dietary Restraint and Disinhibition Are Related to Parental Control in Child Feeding." *Appetite* 35 (2000): 121–129.

CHAPTER 5

In fact, when researchers; When researchers examined: Reedy, J., and S. M. Krebs-Smith. "Dietary Sources of Energy, Solid Fats, and Added Sugars Among Children and Adolescents in the United States." *Journal of the American Dietetic Association* 110, no. 10 (2010): 1477–1484.

You won't be surprised: U.S. Department of Agriculture. U.S. Department of Health and Human Services. *Dietary Guidelines for Americans, 2010.* 7th ed. Washington, DC: U.S. Government Printing Office, 2010.

Did you know: Buzby, J. C., H. F. Wells, and G. Vocke. 2006. "Possible Implications for U.S. Agriculture from Adoption of Select Dietary Guidelines."

U.S. Department of Agriculture. Economic Research Report No. 31. November 2006. ers.usda.gov/media/860109/err31_002.pdf.

Have you heard: NuVal. "Scores." nuval.com/scores.

Have you heard: Smith, J. (marketing director at NuVal). Email discussion with the author, January 2013.

Because public health officials: Fountain, H. "Asked to Get Slim, Cheese Resists." *New York Times*, August 7, 2012, D1.

because cheese is now: Harvard School of Public Health. "Top Food Sources of Saturated Fat in the U.S." In *The Nutrition Source*. hsph.harvard.edu/nutritionsource/top-food-sources-of-saturated-fat-in-the-us.

The USDA recommends: U.S. Department of Agriculture. "Salt." In *Daily Food Plan for Preschoolers*. choosemyplate.gov/preschoolers/daily-food-plans/about-salt.html.

Former U.S. Food and Drug Administration: Kessler, D. A. *The End of Overeating: Taking Control of the Insatiable American Appetite*. New York: Rodale, 2009.

By one estimate: Elliott, C. "Assessing 'Fun Foods': Nutritional Content and Analysis of Supermarket Foods Targeted at Children." *Obesity Reviews*, no. 9 (2008): 368–377.

It doesn't take long: Cornwell, T. B., and A. R. McAlister. "Alternative Thinking About Starting Points in Obesity. Development of Child Taste Preferences." *Appetite* 56 (2011): 428–439.

A pair of researchers: Cornwell, T. B., and A. R. McAlister. "Contingent Choice: Exploring the Relationship Between Sweetened Beverages and Vegetable Consumption." *Appetite* 62, no. 1 (2013): 203–208.

Hmmm: Fox, M. K., E. Condon, R. R. Briefel, et al. "Food Consumption Patterns of Young Preschoolers: Are They Starting Off on the Right Path?" *Journal of the American Dietetic Association* 110, no. 12, suppl. 3 (2010): S52–S59.

While the American Academy of Pediatrics: Wojcicki, J. M., and M. B. Heyman. "Reducing Childhood Obesity by Eliminating 100% Fruit Juice." *American Journal of Public Health* 102, no. 9 (2012): 1630–1633.

Juice has the same: Sell, David. "Dr. Andrew Weil Tells Family Docs: Urge Bans on Soda and Pharmaceutical Advertising." *Philly.Com*, October 18, 2012. philly.com/philly/blogs/phillypharma/Dr-Andrew-Weil-tells-family-docs -Urge-bans-on-soda-and-pharmaceutical-advertising.html.

In the vegetable soup study: Spill, M. K., L. L. Birch, L. S. Roe, and B. J. Rolls. "Serving Large Portions of Vegetable Soup at the Start of Meal Affected Children's Energy and Vegetable Intake." *Appetite* 57 (2011): 213–219.

In the carrot study: Spill, M. K., L. L. Birch, L. S. Roe, and B. J. Rolls. "Eating Vegetables First: The Use of Portion Size to Increase Vegetable Intake in Preschool Children." *American Journal of Clinical Nutrition* 91 (2010): 1237–1243.

A Secret to More Fruit at Breakfast: Harris, J. L., M. B. Schwartz, A. Ustjanauskas, et al. "Effects of Serving High-Sugar Cereals on Children's Breakfast-Eating Behavior." *Pediatrics* 127, no. 1 (2011): 71–76.

CHAPTER 6

Two- to three-year-olds who eat: Nicklaus, S. "Development of Food Variety in Children." *Appetite* 52 (2009): 253–255.

Recent research from Switzerland: van der Horst, K. "Overcoming Picky Eating: Eating Enjoyment as a Central Aspect of Children's Eating Behaviors." *Appetite* 58 (2012): 567–574.

Make "New" Work for You: Pliner, P., and K. Hobden. "Development of a Scale to Measure the Trait of Food Neophobia in Humans." *Appetite* 19 (1992): 105–120.

Research shows that children build up: Dovey, T. M., P. A. Staples, E. L. Gibson, and J. C. G. Halford. "Food Neophobia and 'Picky/Fussy' Eating in Children: A Review." *Appetite* 50 (2008): 181–193.

One study reports a child describing a cauliflower: De Moura, S. L. "Determinants of Food Rejection Amongst School Children." *Appetite* 49 (2007): 716–719.

But research shows that the healthier children think: Wardle, J., and G. Huon. "An Experimental Investigation of the Influence of Health Information on Children's Taste Preferences." *Health Education Research* 15, no. 1 (2000): 39–44.

You can find more ideas: Ernsperger, L., and T. Stegen-Hanson. *Just Take a Bite: Easy, Effective Answers to Food Aversions and Eating Challenges!* Arlington, TX: Future Horizons, 2004.

In a Louisiana State University study: Lakkakula, A., J. Geaghan, M. Zanovec, et al. "Repeated Taste Exposure Increases Liking for Vegetables by Low-Income Elementary School Children." *Appetite* 55 (2010): 226–231.

In another study, English: Wardle, J., L. J. Cooke, E. L. Gibson, et al. "Increasing Children's Acceptance of Vegetables: A Randomized Trial of Parent-Led Exposure." *Appetite* 40 (2003): 155–162.

For instance, in one recent investigation, kids in England: Liem, D. G., L. Zandstra, and A. Thomas. "Prediction of Children's Flavour Preferences: Effect of Age and Stability in Reported Preferences." *Appetite* 55 (2010): 69–75.

A recent study in Mississippi: Thomson, J. L., B. J McCabe-Sellers, E. Strickland, et al. "Development and Evaluation of WillTry: An Instrument for Measuring Children's Willingness to Try Fruits and Vegetables." *Appetite* 54 (2010): 465–472.

You've probably heard: Cooke, L. J., L. C. Chambers, E. V. Añez, and J. Wardle. "Facilitating or Undermining? The Effect of Reward on Food Acceptance: A Narrative Review." *Appetite* 57 (2011): 493–497.

A group of two- to four-year-olds: Horne, P. J., J. Greenhalgh, M. Erjavec, et al. "Increasing Pre-School Children's Consumption of Fruit and Vegetables: A Modelling and Rewards Intervention." *Appetite* 56 (2011): 375–385.

If you want to give rewards: Kazdin, A. E. *The Kazdin Method for Parenting the Defiant Child.* New York: Houghton Mifflin, 2008.

If anxiety is a problem: Nicholls, D., D. Christie, L. Randall, and B. Lask. "Selective Eating: Symptom, Disorder or Normal Variant." *Clinical Child Psychology and Psychiatry* 6, no. 2 (2001): 257–270.

CHAPTER 7

One study documented French mothers: Maier, A., C. Chabanet, B. Schaal, et al. "Food-Related Sensory Experience from Birth Through Weaning: Contrasted Patterns in Two Nearby European Regions." *Appetite* 49 (2007): 429–440.

In both countries: Branum, A. M., and S. L. Lukacs. "Food Allergy Among U.S. Children: Trends in Prevalence and Hospitalizations." NCHS Data Brief No. 10. Hyattsville, MD: National Center for Health Statistics, 2008. cdc.gov/nchs/data/databriefs/db10.pdf.

It turns out that parents: Liem, D. G., L. Zandstra, and A. Thomas. "Prediction of Children's Flavour Preferences: Effect of Age and Stability in Reported Preferences." *Appetite* 55 (2010): 69–75.

A group of third through sixth graders: Mata, J., B. Scheibehenne, and P. M. Todd. "Predicting Children's Meal Preferences: How Much Do Parents Know?" *Appetite* 50 (2008): 367–375.

To find out if the same holds true for children: Capaldi, E. D., and G. J. Privitera. "Decreasing Dislike for Sour and Bitter in Children and Adults." *Appetite* 50 (2008): 139–145.

You can use other preferred flavors: Fraker, C., M. Fishbein, S. Cox, and L. Walbert. *Food Chaining: The Proven 6-Step Plan to Stop Picky Eating, Solve Feeding Problems, and Expand Your Child's Diet.* New York: Marlowe, 2007.

Don't steer clear of challenging: Blossfield, I., A. Collins, M. Kiely, and C. Delahunty. "Texture Preferences of 12-Month-Old Infants and the Role of Early Experiences." *Food Quality and Preference* 18 (2007): 396–404.

Research shows that parents don't: Howard, A. J., K. M. Mallan, R. Byrne, et al. "Toddlers' Food Preferences: The Impact of Novel Food Exposure, Maternal Preferences and Food Neophobia." *Appetite* 59 (2012): 818–825.

In one study of preschool centers: Sweitzer, S. J., M. E. Briley, and C. Robert-Gray. "Do Sack Lunches Provided by Parents Meet the Nutritional Needs of Young Children Who Attend Child Care?" *Journal of the American Dietetic Association* 109, no. 1 (2009): 141–144.

And in another study of school: Johnston, C. A., J. P. Moreno, A. El-Mubasher, and D. Woehler. "School Lunches and Lunches Brought from Home: A Comparative Analysis." *Childhood Obesity* 8, no. 4 (2012): 364–368.

CHAPTER 8

Maybe that's why parents: Laurier, E., and S. Wiggins. "Finishing the Family Meal: The Interactional Organisation of Satiety." *Appetite* 56 (2011): 53–64.

When parents pressure children: Carper, J. L., J. O. Fisher, and L. L. Birch. "Young Girls' Emerging Dietary Restraint and Disinhibition Are Related to Parental Control in Child Feeding." *Appetite* 35 (2000): 121–129.

If you double the amount; When children serve themselves: Fisher, J. O., B. J. Rolls, and L. L. Birch. "Children's Bite Size and Intake of an Entree Are Greater with Large Portions Than with Age-Appropriate or Self-Selected Portions." *American Journal of Clinical Nutrition* 77 (2003): 1164–1170.

It's called our consumption norm; some entrées; You can downsize your kids' consumption: Wansink, B., and K. Van Ittersum. "Portion Size Me: Downsizing Our Consumption Norms." *Journal of the American Dietetic Association* 107, no. 7 (2007): 1103–1106.

the chocolate chip cookie: Young, L. R. *The Portion Teller Plan: The No-Diet Reality Guide to Eating, Cheating, and Losing Weight Permanently.* New York: Three Rivers Press, 2005.

But that makes the situation even worse: Galloway, A. T., L. M. Fiorito, L. A. Francis, and L. L. Birch. "'Finish Your Soup': Counterproductive Effects of Pressuring Children to Eat on Intake and Affect." *Appetite* 46, no. 3 (2006): 318–323.

The Clean Plate Club has a lot of members: Fay, S. H., D. Ferriday, E. C. Hinton, et al. "What Determines Real-World Meal Size? Evidence for Pre-Meal Planning." *Appetite* 56 (2011): 284–289.

The most widely recommended: Satter, E. *How to Get Your Kid to Eat . . . But Not Too Much.* Boulder, CO: Bull, 1987.

Here's a cool way that researchers: Johnson, S. L. "Improving Preschoolers' Self-Regulation of Energy Intake." *Pediatrics* 106, no. 6 (2000): 1429–1435.

Adapted from: Fish, D. *Take the Fight out of Food: How to Prevent and Solve Your Child's Eating Problems.* New York: Atria Books, 2005.

For instance, in addition to Tummy Hunger: Tribole, E., and E. Resch. *Intuitive Eating: A Revolutionary Program That Works.* 2nd ed. New York: St. Martin's Press, 2003.

In his book *Touchpoints*: Brazelton, T. B. *Touchpoints: Your Child's Emotional and Behavioral Development.* Reading, MA: Perseus, 1992.

In 2004, a team of researchers: Mrdjenovic, G., and D. A. Levitsky. "Children Eat What They Are Served: The Imprecise Regulation of Energy Intake." *Appetite* 44, no. 3 (2005): 273–282.

I know that the message: Koletzko, B., and A. M. Toschke. "Meal Patterns and Frequencies: Do They Affect Body Weight in Children and Adolescents?" *Critical Reviews in Food Science and Nutrition* 50 (2010): 100–105.

I know that the message: Newby, P. K. "Are Dietary Intakes and Eating Behaviors Related to Childhood Obesity? A Comprehensive Review of the Evidence." *Journal of Law, Medicine & Ethics* 35, no. 1 (2007): 35–60.

Today's children typically: Piernas, C., and B. M. Popkin. "Trends in Snacking Among U.S. Children." *Health Affairs* 29, no. 3 (2010): 398–404.

When you combine this with the fact: Le Billon, K. *French Kids Eat Everything:*

How Our Family Moved to France, Cured Picky Eating, Banned Snacking, and Discovered 10 Simple Rules for Raising Happy, Healthy Eaters. New York: William Morrow, 2012.

Contentious and unpleasant meals: van der Horst, K. "Overcoming Picky Eating: Eating Enjoyment as a Central Aspect of Children's Eating Behaviors." *Appetite* 58 (2012): 567–574.

When first and sixth graders were offered cookies: Marchiori, D., L. Waroquier, and O. Klein. "'Split Them!' Smaller Item Sizes of Cookies Lead to a Decrease in Energy Intake in Children." *Journal of Nutrition Education and Behavior* 44, no. 3 (2012): 251–255.

That's the kind of prompt: Orrell-Valente, J. K., L. G. Hill, W. A. Brechwald, et al. "'Just Three More Bites': An Observational Analysis of Parents' Socialization of Children's Eating at Mealtime." *Appetite* 48, no. 1 (2007): 37–45.

A 2003 Yale University study: Puhl, R. M., and M. B. Schwartz. "If You Are Good You Can Have a Cookie: How Memories of Childhood Food Rules Link to Adult Eating Behaviors." *Eating Behaviors* 4 (2003): 283–293.

In one classic study: Zimbardo, P., and J. Boyd. *The Time Paradox: The New Psychology of Time That Will Change Your Life.* New York: Free Press, 2008.

They discovered that some people browse: Wansink, B., and C. R. Payne. "Eating Behavior and Obesity at Chinese Buffets." *Obesity* 16, no. 8 (2008): 1957–1960.

CHAPTER 9

Now, however, a study: Brotman, L. M., S. Dawson-McClure, K.-Y. Huang, et al. "Early Childhood Family Interventions and Long-Term Obesity Prevention Among High-Risk Minority Youth." *Pediatrics* 129, no. 3 (2012): e621–e628.

Experts say that most kids: Wallis, D. "Punched and Poked by Their Pride and Joy." *Well* (blog). *New York Times*, May 20, 2013. well.blogs.nytimes.com/2013/05/20/punched-and-poked-by-their-pride-and-joy.

ACKNOWLEDGMENTS

This book was my dream for a very long time, and it would have never become a reality without the help of a number of extraordinary people. I begin by thanking the many families who, over the years, have opened their homes and their hearts to me. Interviewees, clients, and friends: Every lesson in this book can be traced back to what I learned from you.

My heartfelt thanks go to Leigh Ann Hirschman, an exceptional editor. She enthusiastically embraced this book from our very first conversation and worked tirelessly to keep both me and my message on track through some very wordy days. Leigh Ann's guidance and good-natured patience are the reasons this book came together. I am deeply appreciative.

I am indebted to my agent, Betsy Amster, who saw the potential in my rough proposal and quickly became my advocate. I am grateful for Betsy's careful readings of the manuscript; for her continued support; and for her unerring instincts, which always point me in the right direction. My thanks also go out to publisher John Duff and my talented editor, Jeanette Shaw, at Perigee Books for their unstinting commitment to this book.

Tanya Farrell, my first publicist and now my friend, started spreading my message way before there was even a book, and she has never stopped. Tanya turned her family into an eating lab, asking, "What would Dina do?" whenever food questions arose. Fauzia Burke enthusiastically promoted my writing and connected me to the *Huffington Post* and *Psychology Today*.

My friend and neighbor Robin Duerden was my technology mentor. It is to him that I owe my entire online presence. Without Robin there would be no itsnotaboutnutrition.com, no Facebook page, no webinars. There might not even be any email. He has been a sounding board, a strategist, and an emergency technician. (Thanks go to Vickie, too, for patiently lending Robin so often.)

Many thanks to my friends and colleagues, both near and far, online and in person, who provided immeasurable support, good cheer, and good food. Special thanks to Gary Spector for helping me out at the last minute.

And finally, to my amazing family, who surely tired of the endless conversations about food, feeding children, writing challenges, and deadlines but did not show it—words cannot express my gratitude. You provided unending support, lifted me up when I was down, and most important, never let me give up. I am lucky to love you and to be loved by you.

ABOUT THE AUTHOR

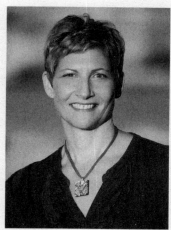

Gary Spector

Dina Rose, PhD, is a sociologist, parent educator, and feeding special-
ist. Trained at Duke University, Dr. Rose worked as a criminologist before she decided to seek out practical, research-based ways to help kids
learn to eat right. She lives in Hoboken, New Jersey, with her husband
and daughter. Join Dr. Rose at her website, itsnotaboutnutrition.com.

It's Not About the Broccoli